# Calculation of Drug Dosages

Caroline Janney, RN, MSN

&

Jane Flahive, BS, MA

Sixth Edition  2003

T J Designs
1237 Laguna Lane
San Luis Obispo, CA 93405
E-mail: DrugCalc@cs.com
Fax: (805) 545-8430

ABOUT THE AUTHORS

Caroline Peterson Janney, R.N., M.S.N.
*Graduate of Henry Ford Community College and*
  *Wayne State University, Michigan*
*Previous Occupations:*
*Instructor of Nursing at:*
*California State University, Long Beach*
*Medical College of Ohio, Toledo*
*Wayne County Community College, Michigan*

Co-author, Jane Flahive, B.S., M.A.
*Graduate of California State University, Long Beach*
*Post Graduate Studies, University of Southern California*
*Previous Occupations:*
*Director, Media Resource Center*
  *California State University, Long Beach*
*Instructional Designer*
  *The Consortium of the California State University*
*Assistant Professor, Nursing Department*
  *California State University, Long Beach*

CREDITS

Design and Production: Carl Schreier, Homestead Publishing, Moose,
  Wyoming and Denver, Colorado.
Photography by King D. Beach, Jr.
Cover photograph by David Friend Productions, San Diego, CA;
  Courtesy of IMED Corporation, San Diego, CA

EDITORIAL

James Flahive, BA, University of North Carolina
Ron Janney, BA, Ohio University

Copyright © 1996 and 2000 by Caroline Peterson Janney.
Sixth Edition. Revised, 2002.
Library of Congress Catalog Card Number 00-090703
ISBN 0-939287-12-9
Printed in China

Co-Author: Chapter Seven: Pediatric Drug Calculation
   Ginger Kee, EdD. RN, Associate Professor University of Texas Houston
Co-Author: Chapter Eight: Intravenous Infusion Rates
   Whei Ming Su, MSN, RN, Associate Professor, Purdue University North Central, Indiana
Co-Author: Chapter Twelve: Dimensional Analysis
   Bonnie Benson, MS, RN, Professor of Nursing, Westminister College, St. Mark's-Westminster School of
   Nursing, Salt Lake City, UT

A Special Thanks to:
Individuals who contributed by editing, being resources, or giving suggestions to improve the book.
   Gen Bahrt, RN, MN, Lecturer, University of California, Los Angeles, CA
   Julie Biner, RN, Critical Care Specialist and Operating Room Specialist, University of Utah, Salt Lake City
   Margaret Brady, PhD., Professor, Nursing, California State University, Long Beach, CA
   Sharon Brown, RN, MN, FNP, California State University, Long Beach, CA
   James Bush, PhD., Professor, Nursing, University of Washington, WA
   Michael Cohen, MS, FASHP, Institute for Safe Medication Practice, Warminster, PA
   Phyllis Crockett, BS R.Ph, St. John's Hospital, Jackson, WY
   Jane Garr, RN, BA, Wheaton College, Norton, MA
   Diane Hayashi, AA, El Camino College, CA
   Ron Karidi, Professor of Mathematics, Stanford Universtiy, Stanford, CA
   Ginger Kee EdD, RN, Associate Professor of Clinical Nursing, University of Texas, TX
   Lisa Knauss, RN, MSN, CCRN, West Chester University, PA
   Jan L. Lee, RN, PhD, CS, Assistant Professor, Universtiy of California, Los Angeles
   Nancy Lischke, Professor of Nursing, San Diego State University, CA
   Marilou Marchetto, BS, R.Ph, St. John's Hospital, Jackson, WY
   Barbara Nelms, California State University, Long Beach, CA
   Beverly J. McClellan, RN, MSN, Assist. Director, ASN Program, Hannibal-Lagrange College, MO
   Linda Robinson, University of New Hampshire, Durham, NH
   Joanne Guyton Simmons, PhD, RN, Medical College of Ohio, Toledo, OH
   Janice Topp, RN. MSN, CNS, Professor of Nursing, Purdue Universtiy North Central, IN
   Dean Ueda, Pharm.D. University of California, Los Angeles, Medical Center, CA
   Paula Vehlow, MS, Southern Illinois University at Edwardsville, IL
   Robin Whittemore, RN, MSN, School of Nursing, University of Conneticut, Storrs, CT
   Joyce S. Willens, PhD, RN, Assistant Professor, College of Nursing, Villanova University, PA

Special thanks to these pharmaceutical companies for their assistance.

| | |
|---|---|
| Abbott Pharmaceuticals | IVAC Corporation |
| A.H. Robbins | Janssen Pharmaceutics |
| American Regert Laboratories Inc. | Lederle Laboratories |
| Astra Pharmaceutical Products | Marion Merrell Dow Inc. |
| Burroughs Wellcome Co. | McNeil Pharmaceuticals |
| DuPont Medical Products | Merck Sharp & Dohme |
| Eli Lilly & Co. | Parke-Davis |
| Elkins Sinn Inc. | Roche Pharmaceuticals |
| Forest Pharmaceuticals Inc. | Roxanne Laboratories |
| Hoffmann La Roche Inc. | Smith Kline & Beecham |
| IMED Corporation | Squibb Managed Health Care Group |

# Comments About the Book

*"Particularly liked the summary tables on the front and back inside covers, clear instructions, and graphics followed by ample drill questions."*

Sister Leona DeBoer
Mount Saint Mary College, New York

*"Material presented from simple to complex and this brings the student immediately into practice situations. Great photos and labels."*

Assistant Professor Janet Brown
California State University, Chico, California

*"I like the way sample problems are provided and the important information is highlighted in the boxes."*

Assistant Professor Patricia Joyce
Washburn University, Kansas

*"Nice to see a good self study book. Thanks."*

North Central Michigan College, Michigan

*"We have found the workbook, Calculation of Drug Dosages to be valuable in teaching the basic principles of drug and IV calculations. It builds from simple to complex and effectively breaks the learning paths into small logical steps. Opportunity to practice at each step facilitates mastery of the content."*

Paula Mobily, PhD, RN
Nursing, University of Iowa

# To the Student

This workbook is designed to make calculating drug dosages easy for you. The workbook uses the Ratio Proportion or Dimensional Analysis methods for calculating most problems and also includes formulas for some problems. The problems in this book are taken from actual clinical situations.

## How to Use the Workbook

Take the Basic Math Review pretest in chapter 14. This pretest will indicate whether you need to study chapter 14, Basic Math Review or begin with chapter 1, Introduction to the Administration of Medications.

This book uses sample problems concerning calculating drug dosages. After each set of sample problems there are practice problems for you to work.

**Chapter 1: Introduction to the Administration of Medication** is divided into six sections.
1. Guidelines for Safe Drug Calculation is based on recent research.
2. The Process of Drug Administration, illustrates the process of administering drugs including interpreting, transcribing, and noting physician's orders. It also includes medications times and records.
3. How to Use the Physician's Desk Reference, illustrates how to look up information on drugs.
4. How to Read Drug Labels, shows actual labels and describes how to read the labels.
5. How Drugs are Supplied, illustrates with photographs various forms of drugs.
6. Equipment Utilized for Drug Administration is depicted and explained. Sample and Practice Problems are included in this chapter.

**Chapter 2: Ratio Proportion**, concerns itself with the ratio proportion method of calculating drug dosages. Sample problems show how to calculate oral and injectable drugs using ratio proportion. Practice problems follow.

**Chapter 3: The Systems of Measure**, explains the metric, apothecary and household systems of measure. Although most drugs are labeled in the metric system, there are some that are still ordered in the apothecary systems of measure. A conversion table is given that should be memorized. When the table is memorized, it is much easier to conceptualize drug calculations.

**Chapter 4: Conversion from One System of Measure to Another**, demonstrates how to convert from apothecary to metric and how to convert within the metric system using the decimal method. Sample problems are followed by practice problems on conversions.

**Chapter 5: Drug Calculation Requiring Conversions**, concerns itself with drug calculations that require conversions and shows how to change the physician's order into the same units in which the medication is supplied. Read the sample problem and work the practice problems.

**Chapter 6: Reconstitution of Powdered Drugs**, explains why drugs are stored in powdered form, how to reconstitute the drugs, and how to fill out the label correctly after reconstituting. After reading the chapter, you should be able to read a label and reconstitute a drug.

**Chapter 7: Pediatric Drug Calculation**, explains the nurse's responsibility in administering pediatric dosages, shows how to round off dosages, how to determine if the dosage is safe, how to calculate pediatric dosages, and how to determine a child's body-surface area based on the West Nomogram Chart. Practice problems follow each section to ensure your understanding of the concepts.

**Chapter 8: Intravenous Infusion Rates, discusses** general concepts in administering fluids, blood and total parenteral nutrition. The nurses responsibility in this process is explained. Sample problems demonstrate how to calculate drops per minute and how to calculate intravenous infusion rates using a pump. Practice problems follow each concept.

**Chapter 9: Heparin,** gives general information about why Heparin is used, how to calculate the intravenous flow rates with sample problems and concludes with practice problems.

**Chapter 10: Insulin Drug Calculation,** includes a description of insulin, the sources of insulin, the units, the syringes, how to measure correct dosages, how to mix two insulins in the same syringe and nursing responsibilities in regard to insulin. Practice problems follow the concepts.

**Chapter 11: Titrated Drugs Used in Critical Care Settings,** has content that may not be required as a part of the nursing curriculum. However, it is a reference for nurses working in specialty areas. Included in the chapter are: Hints for safe IV drug calculation, how to use an electronic infusion pump to titrate potent vasopressor drugs, sample problems and practice problems.

**Chapter 12: Community Nursing and the Elderly,** discusses patient teaching in the home care setting with emphasis on medications and the elderly. Sample and practice problems are given for preparing a weaker solution from a stock solution. Lastly, elderly drug dosage based on body weight and/or creatinine clearance using the Crockrof-Gault Formula is presented.

**Chapter 13: Dimensional Analysis,** is another method of doing drug calculation. It is included as a separate chapter so that it is not confused with the proportion method. Sample problems of each type of drug calculation are given using the dimensional analysis method. The student is referred to the appropriate practice problems in other chapters.

**Chapter 14: Basic Math Review,** presents a basic review of Roman numerals, decimals and fractions. After reviewing the content you will be able to recognize the values of Roman Numerals, add, subtract, multiply and divide decimals and fractions and find equivalents of decimals, fractions, ratios and percents. This chapter is for students who feel they need assistance in basic math skills. It is not intended for all students.

In summary, it is the intent of this book to make drug dosage calculations easier for you. As mentioned previously, this workbook utilizes the Ratio Proportion and Dimensional Analysis methods, which were selected because they can be used for different types of problems in drug dosage calculations. Both methods reduce learning many rules that tend to be confusing.

Be sure to examine each Sample Problem in the book. The answers to the Practice Problems in each section can be found at the end of each chapter or in some cases the answers will follow the problems. Commonly used abbreviations are found on the inside front cover and common conversions can be found on the inside back cover. Chapter 13 utilizes an alternate method called Dimensional Analysis. Some students may prefer this method, as it is often used in chemistry and physics courses.

After studying the chapters, doing the practice problems and checking your answers, you may want to take a Post Test. The Post Test is located in the back of chapter 13. The Post Test will indicate your knowledge level on calculating and administering drug dosages.

# Objectives

Upon completion of chapters 1-13, you will be able to:

Explain the process of drug administration.

Use the ratio proportion method to calculate drug dosages.

Convert one system of measurement to another.

Calculate drug dosages that require conversions.

Reconstitute powdered drugs.

Calculate drug dosages for infants and children.

Determine the drip rate for intravenous medication.

Calculate drug dosages for Heparin.

Measure insulin correctly.

Use formulas to titrate potent vasopressor drugs in critical care settings.

Mix a weaker solution from a stock solution.

Calculate an estimated creatinine clearance using Crockrof-Gault formula.

Determine safe dosages for the elderly.

Perform patient teaching in the home setting.

## Basic Math Skills
See Chapter Fourteen

If you need a refresher on basic math skills and complete chapter 14, you will be able to do basic math skills such as adding, subtracting, multiplying, and dividing decimals and fractions. Additionally, you will be able to find equivalents for decimals, fractions, ratios and percents.

## Reference Book
Save this book as a reference for unforeseen changes in clinical practice. The index provides a quick reference to methods and formulas for drug calculations. Some areas of clinical practice require few drug calculations, whereas other areas of practice require numerous calculations.

# Table of Contents

# Table of Contents

# Table of Contents

1

Chapter One

# Introduction

to the

# Administration

of

# Medication

| Physician's Order Sheet | | |
|---|---|---|
| Date | Time | |
| 9/14 | 8 am | Demerol 35 mg IM q4h prn for pain<br><br>*Dr. Smith* |
| Date<br>9/14 | Time<br>8:15 am | Noted    C Jones R.N. |

Give

Fig. 1

## Available from the Pharmacy

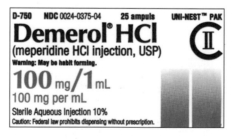

Demerol 100 mg in 1 mL

Fig. 2

# The nurse must calculate the correct dosage

RATIO PROPORTION METHOD

$$\frac{35 \text{ mg}}{X \text{ mL}} = \frac{100 \text{ mg}}{1 \text{ mL}}$$

$$100 X = 35$$

$$X = 0.35$$

*See Chapter 2*

**Fig. 3**

Observe medical asepsis before preparing medications by washing your hands. Check to see if the patient has any allergies before administering drugs.

DIMENSIONAL ANALYSIS METHOD

$$\frac{35 \text{ mg}}{1} \times \frac{1 \text{ mL}}{100 \text{ mg}} = \underline{\hspace{1cm}} \text{ mL}$$

$$\frac{35 \text{ mL}}{100} = 0.35 \text{ mL}$$

*See Chapter 13*

**Fig. 4**

The drawings illustrate part of the process of drug administration. The nurse determines from the physician's order sheet that the patient may receive Demerol 35 mg prn every four hours for pain (Fig. 1). Demerol is a narcotic, which is a controlled substance kept locked in the narcotic drawer. The nurse obtains the Demerol and then reads the label carefully. Fig. 2 shows 100 mg of Demerol in 1 mL of solution. The nurse wishes to give 35 mg from the 100 mg. What part of 1 mL contains 35 mg? Fig. 3 illustrates the Ratio Proportion method for calculation of the dosage found in chapter 2. Fig. 4 demonstrates the Dimensional Analysis method for calculation of the dosage found in chapter 13. Thirty-five one hundredths of 1 mL contains 35 mg. The nurse finds the 0.35 mL mark on the syringe and draws 0.35 mL into the syringe. The remaining 0.65 mL of excess solution is discarded. Use a tuberculin syringe to measure 0.35 mL (see page 36). When an excess amount of narcotic is discarded, the nurse must co-sign the narcotic sheet with another nurse who has witnessed the process.

**Note:** *Choose one method for drug calculation, either Ratio Proportion or Dimensional Analysis. Occasionally a formula may be preferable to either of the above methods.*

# Introduction

The illustrations on pages 2 & 3 show part of the process of administering drugs. This chapter is divided into sections that are important to administering medications correctly and safely. First, Guidelines for Safe Drug Calculation, including the five rights of drug administration. Second, The Process of Drug Administration including the physicians order sheet, interpretation of the order, transcription of the order to the Medication Administration Record and Kardex, and military time schedules. Third, How to Use the Physician's Desk Reference. Fourth, Reading Drug Labels. Fifth, How Drugs Are Supplied. Sixth, Equipment Utilized for Drug Dosage Measurement.

## Guidelines for Safe Drug Calculation

Despite the emphasis of the five rights of drug administration, far too many patients receive the wrong medication. According to Gayle Hacker Sullivan, RN JD, medication errors are among the ten most common allegations in nursing liability cases.

Medication errors have occurred throughout the history of nursing. The headline in the "Rocky Mountain News" dated November 14, 1993 stated, *Medication Errors Kept Secret*. This was followed with a subhead which read," Life threatening mistakes repeated because hospitals don't share information". The article goes on to state that every day patients are given the wrong medicine or the wrong dose, and that the same errors are repeated again and again.

To help insure the proper delivery of drugs we present the following suggestions:

### The Patient's Bill of Rights

Besides having the normal rights of life, liberty and the pursuit of happiness, a patient has five additional rights concerning the administration of drugs which are:

> **THE FIVE RIGHTS**
>
> The Right Drug
> The Right Dosage
> The Right Patient
> The Right Time
> The Right Route

### The Right Drug

Although all of the rights are very important, the administration of the correct drug has to be considered paramount. The nurse must take every precaution to ensure that the proper drug is administered.

One of the most common errors is caused by the nurse misreading the drug order or by misreading the label. There is an increasing number of drug names that are very similar and can easily be mistaken for each other, especially when handwritten. The following is a list of some of these drugs.

| LOOK ALIKE DRUGS | | | |
|---|---|---|---|
| amiodarone | amrinone | hydralazine | hydroxyzine |
| aminophylline | ampicillin | norfloxacin | Norflex |
| Banthine | Brethine | Roxanol | Roxicet |
| Celebrex | Celexa | Halcion | Haldol |
| Doxidan | Doriden | Xanax | Zantac |

**The Right Drug** *cont.*

The list is a small sampling of look alike drugs that can easily be misinterpreted with scrawled handwriting. If you can not read the order, do not assume anything. Take the time to confirm the order with the physician. Have the physician spell the order and state why the drug was ordered. When you are sure that you have the proper drug, proceed with the administration.

A more subtle example is the case of a patient who received a prescription for norfloxacin which was prescribed to combat a persistent fever and urinary track infection. The family of the patient noticed that her condition was not improving and that her gait was unsteady. She was referred to a specialist in infectious diseases. The specialist reviewed the patient's current medications and discovered that she was taking Norflex, a muscle relaxant rather than the prescribed drug. The pharmacist had misread the prescription.

This illustrates how poor handwriting and look alike drugs can lead to serious mistakes. Always read the labels carefully, never assume anything, and when in doubt, find out for sure.

An article appeared in the Jackson Hole Daily Guide on November 18, 1999, about electronic prescription pads. The electronic prescription pad, used by an increasing number of physicians, is one solution to poor handwriting and look alike drugs. With a few clicks, the physician can e-mail the prescription directly to the drug store or pharmacy. Electronic prescribing started in hospitals, where doctors leave a patient's bedside to type prescriptions on a special computer at the nursing station. The Journal of the American Medical Association reported last year that such computerized prescriptions cut by more than half the rate of serious medication errors at one hospital. The pharmacist can easily determine Celebrex from Celexa from Cerebyx.

**Confirmation Bias**

Confirmation bias occurs when the nurse looks for what is familiar such as the **color and shape of a vial,** and satisfied that he or she knows what the vial contains, fails to read the label.

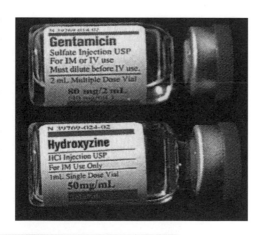

As you can see with the illustration, it would be very easy to mistake gentamicin for hydroxyzine if the nurse did not read the label. This also occurred when a nurse administered a bolus of potassium chloride instead of 5 mL of normal saline. The nurse chose the vial by color and size, rather than by reading the label. This haste caused serious consequences. This could have been easily avoided if the nurse had thought to remember the basic procedure for reading the label three times before administering the drug.

> **READ THE LABEL THREE TIMES**
> 1. Read the label when you first pick up the vial.
> 2. Read the label after you have drawn the medication into the syringe.
> 3. Read the label again before you discard the vial or return it to the drawer.

A mistake that prompted the Board of Registered Nurses in the State of California to issue a practice alert was that potassium chloride was administered rather than Lasix. Their report in 1993 found that of nineteen disciplinary actions against RN licenses between October 1987 and February 1992, five involved the mistaken substitution of KCl for Lasix. It was further decided that these errors usually occur in settings where nurses are expected to function rapidly. The error may have been in not reading the label, or drawing KCl and Lasix into separate syringes and then not labeling the syringes.

## Confirmation Bias *Cont*

Do not store KCl and Lasix in the same area, and be sure to label drugs drawn into syringes carefully. Another area of confirmation bias can occur with pre-mixed intravenous solutions.

A nurse in a cath lab hung a bag of D5W with 2 g of Lidocaine pre-mixed in the solution assuming that it was plain D5W. The nurse did not read the label completely. This error was discovered before it caused serious complications for the patient.

In a perfect world no one would store pre-mixed IV solutions in the same area as plain IV solutions. If you are ever in a work place that keeps them together, take the time to read the label three times before administering any drug or hanging any IV. Present suggestions for changes to your supervisor.

As you have read this section it must have become obvious to you that errors in drug administration are always avoidable if proper care and time are taken. Although excuses can always be given in a situation ("I was in a hurry..., There was too much to do..., We are short staffed.") there really is no excuse. Too much is at stake when it comes to administering drugs. Always read the labels carefully, never assume anything, and when in doubt, find out for sure.

## The Right Dosage

When administering a drug, the nurse is legally and morally responsible to calculate and administer the right dosage. Even though the nurse on the shift preceding yours may have calculated the dosage and administered it without any noticeable ill effects, you are responsible from the moment you come on shift. You do not want to continue with an improper dosage, and you will not know for sure whether or not it is, in fact, calculated correctly until you calculate it yourself. Do not administer any medication until you are sure the dosage is correct. Clear handwriting and accurate transcription are critical in preventing drug errors. Take the time to write clearly and legibly.

Always precede a decimal with a zero. Do not place a decimal point after a whole number.

| DO WRITE | DO NOT WRITE |
|----------|--------------|
| 0.1 g | .1 g  This could be mistaken for 1 g |
| 1 g | 1.0 g  This could be mistaken for 10 |

It is not necessary to point out the critical situation that could arise from either of these two simple errors.

> ### THE RIGHT DOSAGE
> Always calculate the dosage yourself before administering any drug.
> Always take time to write clearly and legibly.
> Always precede a decimal with a zero and never use a decimal after a whole number.
> Always double check calculations with another nurse, if in doubt.

## The Right Patient

The patient has the right to receive the medicine that has been prescribed for his specified illness. For that reason always identify the patient before administering any medication. Ask the patient for his or her name and verify it with the arm band. There is a reason for double checking. The patient may not have heard you correctly, or answered to the wrong name. It may seem like a waste of time, but consider the consequences if a mistake is made.

Whenever a patient questions the drug that is about to be administered, do not hesitate to double check the order. Many patients are well informed as to what drug they should be receiving and their observations may prevent an error.

> BEFORE ADMINSTERING ANY MEDICATION:
> 1. Ask the patient for his or her name.
> 2. Verify patient's name with the armband.
> 3. Check the patient's name against the MAR which you used as the guide to prepare your medication.

## The Right Route

The right route for each drug should be specified in the physician's order. Safe dosages are established for different routes of administration based on rates of absorption. For example, an order may have been written for a patient to receive morphine by mouth and later the order is changed to receive it intravenously. The dosage for rapidly absorbed intravenous morphine is not the same as the more slowly absorbed oral morphine. When the route is changed, the dosage must be changed accordingly.

Routes of drug administration are not interchangeable. All orders for medications must specify the route. As with all other drugs, be sure to read the label carefully in order to confirm that it is labeled for the intended route. For example, the label on a container of eye drops should always state that the contents of the container are for ophthalmic use. Likewise, the label on the container for ear drops should state that the contents of the container are for otic use.

Document all injection sites on the medication record.

## The Right Time

It is essential to follow a regular schedule when giving medications. A regular schedule helps to maintain a therapeutic blood level of the drug. Medications should be given within 30 minutes either way of the time scheduled. The medication time schedule selected by the hospital should be followed since there is less chance of omission when the drug is given according to schedule.

> MEDICATION TIME SCHEDULE
> 1. Follow the prescribed medication schedule.
> 2. Give the medication within 30 minutes before or after the scheduled time.
> 3. Give the medications before, after, or during meals as required.

## Working Conditions: Staffing

Sufficient staffing and ample time to administer medications should be provided. This helps to prevent fatigue, and avoid carelessness when administering medications.

The preparation of drugs should be done in an area which is free from interruptions and distractions. When performing this most critical of tasks, no one should be disturbed by telephones, orders, or various conversations. The work place should provide this type of setting for the preparation of medications.

## Verbal Orders

Though preferable, it is not always possible for drug orders to be in a written form. The reasons for this are varied, and sometimes are unavoidable, but verbal orders should be discouraged as much as possible. Whether the verbal order is given in person or on the telephone, it is easy to hear the drug incorrectly because there is a similarity in the names of some medications.

If receiving a verbal order is unavoidable, you should insist on the following steps. First of all, make sure that the physician dictates the order slowly and clearly. This accomplished, the nurse should repeat the order back, so that the physician may verify that it has been communicated properly and taken down correctly. Then, within twenty-four hours, the order must be signed by the physician.

> ### VERBAL ORDERS
> 1. Have physician dictate the order clearly and slowly.
> 2. Repeat the order back to the physician to verify.

Occasionally, it will be necessary for the nurse to call in an order to the pharmacist for a drug that is needed immediately. The above procedure must be followed to insure proper communication. If it is possible, a fax sent to the pharmacist is preferable with the order faxed directly to the pharmacy department. When the drug is received, read the label carefully in order to ensure that it is the drug that was ordered.

Taking a few precautions can reduce the risk of verbal orders. However, verbal orders should be avoided whenever possible due to the fact that verbal orders side step some of the checks and balances of the medication delivery system. However, you are the final check and balance in the system. Never assume anything and when in doubt find out for sure.

## Education

It goes without saying, that education in the proper administration of drugs is essential if the nurse is to become sufficiently informed concerning the drugs he or she will be expected to administer on a regular basis. There are so many different drugs presently in use that at times the process of remembering all of their uses and methods of delivery may be overwhelming. Education is the key to competency in the administration of drugs.

The nurse is expected to complete and pass a class in drug calculation. After learning about drugs and showing a theoretical proficiency with them, the nurse, through repeated experience in the field, will become more aware of the various drugs and the proper method of administration. In most situations this would represent sufficient training. However, in the hospital setting one experiences conditions that are considered specialized. Each area of specialization has certain drugs which are used on a regular basis. After working in specialized areas, the nurse becomes very familiar with the drugs that are most often used.

## Education *cont.*

For example, nurses in a Coronary Care Unit administer many cardiovascular drugs while oncology nurses administer chemotherapeutic drugs. Although, as a professional, you are expected to be flexible there is much to be said for repetitive familiarity. For this reason, if you find yourself in an area with which you have a minimal background, you will need to receive some specialized education before you risk a dangerous situation. If there is time and opportunity, adequate staff orientation should be all that is necessary for you to be able to work with drugs in a specialized unit. However, if proper orientation is impossible due to the temporary nature of the present assignment (floated) then it is important that you inform the charge nurse of the float unit of your knowledge base and request that the unit's permanent nurse administer the medications. If the administration plans to send you to this unit on a more frequent basis, then you should request cross training. Whatever the case, always read the labels carefully, never assume anything, and when in doubt, find out for sure.

Neil Davis and Michael Cohen, have started the Institute for Safe Medication Practices. This includes a drug hot line where errors can be reported. Data is tracked, and publicized so health professionals can learn from one another's mistakes. The drug hot line number is 1 800 23 ERROR. Dr. Cohen writes a regular column in "Nursing 2001". He collects and publishes data regarding drug errors. The findings have been instrumental in helping to prevent errors and have been the cause of changes in labeling and packaging by drug companies.

## References:

Board of Registered Nurses, California Board of Registered Nurses Report, Winter, 1993.

Sullivan, Gayle Hacker RN, JD. *Legally Speaking, Five rights equal 0 errors.* "RN Magazine". June, 1991 p65-66.

*Medication Errors Kept Secret.* "Rocky Mountain News". Nov 14, 1993.
Michael Cohen PHARM D. M.S., FASHP and Neil Davis, PHARM D. M.S., FASHP Institute for Safe Medication Practice, 320 W Street Rd. Warminster, PA 18974.

# The Process of Drug Administration

## The Physician's Order

As stated, the illustrations on pages 2 and 3 show part of the process of administering medications to the patient. The doctor sees the patient and then writes the orders on the Physician's Order Sheet. Medication orders must contain all of the following information for each drug.

Examine the order sheet

| PHYSICIAN'S ORDER SHEET | | | |
|---|---|---|---|
| **Date** | **Time** | **Orders** | **Patient Name** |
| | | | Mary Jones |
| | | | 372-04-0865 |
| 3/5 __ | 0900 | DX - Congestive heart failure (CHF) | |
| | | Bed rest with BRP | |
| | | Lanoxin 0.25 mg po qd | |
| | | Bumex 2 mg po qd | |
| | | Potassium Chloride sol 20 mEq po tid | |
| | | Isordil 30 mg po q8h | |
| | | Omnipen -N  1 g IV PB q6h | |
| | | morphine sulfate 2 mg IV q3 h prn chest pain | |
| | | 500 mL D5W KVO | |
| **TIME NOTED** | | **NURSES SIGNATURE** | **DOCTORS SIGNATURE** |
| 3/5 | 0945 | J. Biner, RN | Dr. Lurie |
| **Date** | **Time** | **Orders** | **Patient Name** |
| 3/5 ___ | 0900 | | Mary Jones |
| | | | 372-04-0865 |
| | | Dalmane 15 mg po HS prn sleep | |
| | | I&O | |
| | | 2 g Sodium diet | |
| | | Weigh q AM | |
| | | Chest XR in AM | |
| | | Lytes in AM | |
| | | Digoxin level in AM | |
| | | Call if chest pain unrelieved by Morphine | |
| | | VS q4h | |
| **TIME NOTED** | | **NURSES SIGNATURE** | **DOCTORS SIGNATURE** |
| 3/5 | 0945 | J. Biner, RN | Dr. Lurie |
| | | PLEASE USE BALL POINT PEN ONLY | |

## Interpretation of a Physician's Orders

This is one example of orders written by a physician. Each order contains abbreviations as a part of the order. Refer to the abbreviations on the inside front cover of the book. To read and interpret an order, the abbreviations must be understood.

# Interpretation of Physician's Orders and Abreviations

■ *Lanoxin 0.25 mg po qd means:*

Answer: Give Lanoxin 0.25 mg (milligrams) po (per os or by mouth) qd (everyday)

Use the abbreviations on the inside front cover and write what each order means.

1. DX - Congestive heart failure (CHF)

2. Bed rest with BRP

3. Bumex 2 mg po qd

4. Potassium Chloride sol 20 mEq po tid

5. Isordil 30 mg po q8h

6. Omnipen-N 1 g   IV PB q6h

7. morphine sulfate 2 mg  IV q3h prn chest pain

8. 500 mL of D5W KVO

9. Dalmane 15 mg po  HS prn sleep

10. I&O

11. 2 g Sodium diet

12. Weigh q AM

13. Chest XR in AM

14. Lytes in AM

15. Digoxin level in AM

16. Call if chest pain is unrelieved by Morphine

17. VS q4h

Answers: Chapter 1, 1-17

1. Dx - Diagnosis 2. Activity is bed rest with bathroom privileges only. 3. Give Bumex 2 milligrams per mouth everyday. 4. Give Potassium Chloride solution 20 milliequivalents by mouth three times per day. 5. Give Isordil 30 milligrams by mouth every 8 hours. 6. Give Omnipen-N 1 gram intravenously, diluted in 50 mL of 5 % Dextrose and water, to run piggyback to the main intravenous line every 6 hours. 7. Give morphine sulfate 2 milligrams intravenously every 3 hours when necessary for chest pain. 8. Run 500 milliliters of 5% Dextrose and water, to keep vein open. This means the IV is run at about 10 milliliters per hour to prevent the line from clotting off. 9. Give Dalmane 15 milligrams every bedtime when needed for patient to sleep. 10. Record intake and output every shift. 11. Order a 2 g Sodium Diet for the patient. 12. Weigh the patient every morning. 13. Order chest x-ray for tomorrow morning. 14. Order serum electrolytes for tomorrow morning. 15. Order serum Digoxin level for tomorrow morning. 16. Call Dr. Lurie to report chest pain is not relieved by Morphine. 17. Take vital signs every 4 hours.

# The Process of Drug Administration *cont.*

## Transcription of Orders

The charts with orders must be flagged by the physician, indicating that there are new orders on the chart to be transcribed and noted. The method of flagging a chart varies from one medical center to another. It is very important, no matter what method of flagging is used, that the charts should not be put back in the rack without indicating that there are changes in the orders.

It is the unit secretary's responsibility to read and transcribe the order to the patient's Medication Administration Record. When a Kardex is used, the unit secretary also transcribes the order to the Kardex in pencil.

The physician's order must be written with a ballpoint pen that goes through to the carbonless copy.
The carbonless copy of the order is sent to the pharmacy to be filled. This makes it possible for the pharmacist to read the original order. This method ensures that both the pharmacist and the nurse have checked the original order. This redundancy, which is built into the system, provides another safeguard for patient safety.

## Noting Medication Orders

After the unit secretary transcribes the order onto the Medication Administration Record and the Kardex, the nurse checks the unit secretary's work and approves its correctness by signing his/her name, the time that it was approved, and duly noted. The nurse needs to check the following: 1. That all aspects of the drug order have been transcribed accurately; 2. The handwriting is legible; 3. Zeros precede decimal points; 4. Zeros do not follow decimal points.

## The Kardex

Since the advent of the computer generated Medication Administration Record (MAR), the Kardex is no longer standard on every unit. On units such as Day Surgery, the patients have few orders compared to long term patients. In these instances the Kardex is double the work of transcription. With short term patients it is very simple to verify the MAR with the original physician's order. However, the Kardex is a valuable asset on units with long term patients. General drugs are current for 30 days unless there is an order to the contrary. This means that to check the current MAR, it would be necessary to go through thirty days of physician's orders, a very time consuming task. Each time an order is written, it is transcribed onto the patient's Kardex in pencil. When a drug order is discontinued, it is erased from the Kardex.

Special orders can be clearly spelled out on the Kardex. Suppose a patient is on a reducing schedule of Decadron—a steroid that cannot be stopped abruptly. This reducing schedule can be written on the Kardex so the nurse can quickly check to ascertain what the scheduled dosage is on any given day. If the Kardex is used, the current MAR should be compared with the Kardex checking to be sure all drugs are listed correctly on the MAR at the beginning of every shift. If the MAR is incorrect, double check the Kardex with the original physician's order. When the computer generated MAR is incorrect, notify the pharmacy of the discrepancies. All charts should be checked once a shift for new orders. This is a safeguard to prevent omission of new orders.

## Medication Time Schedule

Medication time schedules can vary from one hospital to another. You must become familiar with the time schedule of the unit on which you are working. Most hospitals use military time to avoid confusion with the AM and PM medication times. Military time is based on a 24 hour clock. Below are two clocks comparing military time with the AM and PM clock. Military time begins at 0100 (1 AM) and ends at 2400 (midnight).

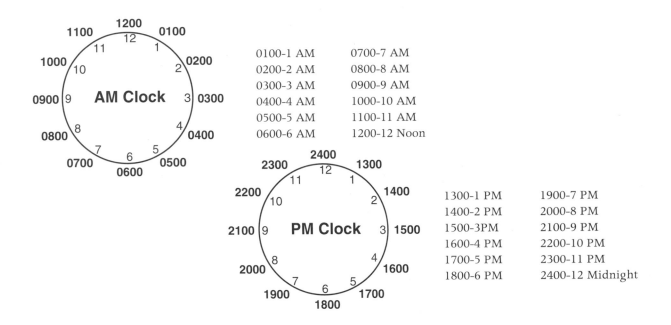

| 0100-1 AM | 0700-7 AM |
|---|---|
| 0200-2 AM | 0800-8 AM |
| 0300-3 AM | 0900-9 AM |
| 0400-4 AM | 1000-10 AM |
| 0500-5 AM | 1100-11 AM |
| 0600-6 AM | 1200-12 Noon |

| 1300-1 PM | 1900-7 PM |
|---|---|
| 1400-2 PM | 2000-8 PM |
| 1500-3PM | 2100-9 PM |
| 1600-4 PM | 2200-10 PM |
| 1700-5 PM | 2300-11 PM |
| 1800-6 PM | 2400-12 Midnight |

## Medication Time Schedules A & B

Listed below are two frequently used time schedules.

| | | Schedule A | | | | Schedule B | | | |
|---|---|---|---|---|---|---|---|---|---|
| bid | twice a day | 0900 | 1700 | | | 1000 | 1800 | | |
| tid | three times a day | 0900 | 1300 | 1700 | | 1000 | 1400 | 1800 | |
| qid | four times a day | 0900 | 1300 | 1700 | 2100 | 1000 | 1400 | 1800 | 2200 |
| q4h | every four hours | 0900 | 1300 | 1700 | | 1000 | 1400 | 1800 | |
| | | 2100 | 0100 | 0500 | | 2200 | 0200 | 0600 | |
| q6h | every six hours | 0900 | 1500 | 2100 | 0300 | 0600 | 1200 | 1800 | 2400 |
| q8h | every eight hours | 0600 | 1400 | 2200 | | 0700 | 1500 | 2300 | |
| qhs | at bedtime | 2100 | | | | 2200 | | | |
| ac | before meals | 0700 | 1100 | 1600 | | 0700 | 1100 | 1600 | |
| pc | after meals | 0900 | 1300 | 1700 | | 1000 | 1400 | 1800 | |

**Convert regular time to military time.**

18. 1 AM  _____

19. 3 AM  _____

20. 12 Noon  _____

21. 6 AM  _____

22. 6 PM  _____

23. 9 AM  _____

24. 7:30PM  _____

25. 2 PM  _____

26. 10 PM  _____

27. 4 PM  _____

**Convert military time to regular time.**

28. 0200  _____

29. 1300  _____

30. 0400  _____

31. 2000  _____

32. 0715  _____

33. 2130  _____

34. 2400  _____

35. 1000  _____

36. 1530  _____

37. 2300  _____

Answers: Chapter 1, 18-27

| 18. 0100 | 21. 0600 | 24. 1930 | 27. 1600 |
| 19. 0300 | 22. 1800 | 25. 1400 | |
| 20. 1200 | 23. 0900 | 26. 2200 | |

Answers: Chapter 1, 28-37

| 28. 2 AM | 31. 8 PM | 34. midnight | 37. 11 PM |
| 29. 1 PM | 32. 7:15 AM | 35. 10 AM | |
| 30. 4 AM | 33. 9:30 PM | 36. 3:30 PM | |

# Medication Administration Record

Practice transcribing the following medications to the Medication Administration Record. Use schedule B for the medication times. In clinical practice the MAR is written in ink. After transcribing to the MAR, transcribe all the orders to the Kardex. Usually the nurse notes the orders and the secretary transcribes. However, there are times the nurse assumes this task.

Examine the order sheet

| PHYSICIAN'S ORDER SHEET | | | |
|---|---|---|---|
| **Date** | **Time** | **Orders** | **Patient Name** |
| | | | Mary Jones |
| | | | 372-04-0865 |
| 3/5 ___ | 0900 | *DX - Congestive heart failure (CHF)* | |
| | | *Bed rest with BRP* | |
| | | *Lanoxin 0.25 mg po qd* | |
| | | *Bumex 2 mg po qd* | |
| | | *Potassium Chloride sol 20 mEq po tid* | |
| | | *Isordil 30 mg po q8h* | |
| | | *Omnipen -N 1 g IV PB q6h* | |
| | | *morphine sulfate 2 mg IV q3 h prn chest pain* | |
| | | *500 mL D5W KVO* | |
| **TIME NOTED** | | **NURSES SIGNATURE** | **DOCTORS SIGNATURE** |
| *3/5* | *0945* | *J. Biner, RN* | *Dr. Lurie* |
| **Date** | **Time** | **Orders** | **Patient Name** |
| 3/5 ___ | 0900 | | Mary Jones |
| | | | 372-04-0865 |
| | | *Dalmane 15 mg po HS prn sleep* | |
| | | *I&O* | |
| | | *2 g Sodium diet* | |
| | | *Weigh q AM* | |
| | | *Chest XR in AM* | |
| | | *Lytes in AM* | |
| | | *Digoxin level in AM* | |
| | | *Call if chest pain unrelieved by Morphine* | |
| | | *VS q4h* | |
| **TIME NOTED** | | **NURSES SIGNATURE** | **DOCTORS SIGNATURE** |
| *3/5* | *0945* | *J. Biner, RN* | *Dr. Lurie* |
| | | PLEASE USE BALL POINT PEN ONLY | |

Mary Jones is 69 years old, weighs 110 pounds, and is currently in room 445. She is allergic to sulfa.

**Owen Healthcare, Inc.**

MEDICATION ADMINISTRATION RECOR[D]

| PHYSICIAN | | PT. WT. | PT. AGE. |
|---|---|---|---|
| SPECIAL REMARKS | | | |
| DIAGNOSIS | | | |
| ALLERGIES | | | |

PAGE_____ OF _____

| LOCATION CODES | ANT. THIGH | GLUTEAL REGION | DELTOID MUSCLE | VENTRAL GLUTEAL | ABDOMINAL | UPPER ARM |
|---|---|---|---|---|---|---|
| | RIGHT - B | RIGHT - D | RIGHT - F | RIGHT - H | RIGHT - K | RIGHT - R |
| | LEFT - C | LEFT - E | LEFT - G | LEFT - J | LEFT - L | LEFT - S |

| SCHEDULED MEDICATIONS | | | | | | | | |
|---|---|---|---|---|---|---|---|---|
| START | STOP | MEDICATION-DOSAGE-FREQUENCY-ROUTE | TIME | DATE | DATE | DATE | DATE | DATE |
| | | | | | | | | |
| | | | | | | | | |
| | | | | | | | | |

| PRN MEDICATIONS | | | | SINGLE ORDERS AND PRE-OPS | | |
|---|---|---|---|---|---|---|
| INITIALS | FULL SIGNATURE | TITLE | DATE | MEDICATION-DOSAGE-ROUTE | TIME | INITIAL[S] |
| | | | | | | |
| | | | | | | |

| ROOM | PATIENT NAME | AM | PM |
|---|---|---|---|

M | 1 | 2 | 3 | 4 | 5 | 6 | 7 | 8 | 9 | 10 | 11 | N | 1 | 2 | 3 | 4 | 5 | 6 | 7 | 8 | 9 | 10 |

ALLERGIES

| DATE | MEDICATIONS | | DATE | IV'S | | DATE | LAB | | DATE | MISCELLANEOUS |
|---|---|---|---|---|---|---|---|---|---|---|
| | | | | | | | | | DATE | X-RAY |

| DATE | RESPIRATORY THERAPY | | DATE | TREATMENTS & PROCEDURES |
|---|---|---|---|---|

| DATE | VITAL SIGNS | DATE | PCMS✓s |
|---|---|---|---|
| | I/O | S/A | S/G |
| | DIET | | |

| DATE | ACTIVITY |
|---|---|

CHRONIC MED. PROBLEM

EMERGENCY NOTIFICATION

PHYSICIAN         CONSULT         ADM. DIAG.

SURGERY PROCEDURE

HOSP. #         ROOM #         NAME:

SEX:  M   F   ADMIT TIME

AGE:         ADMIT DATE

SJ 60285 · REV 11/91

Owen Healthcare, Inc.

MEDICATION ADMINISTRATION RECORD

MARY JONES
Room 445

372 040865

| PHYSICIAN | Lurie | PT. WT. 110 | PT. AGE. 69 |
| SPECIAL REMARKS | | | |
| DIAGNOSIS | CHF | | |
| ALLERGIES | SULFA | | |

OHI-328 Copyright 2/81 (Rev. 5/94)
Owen Healthcare, Inc. All Rights Reserved
PAGE _1_ OF _1_

| LOCATION CODES | ANT. THIGH RIGHT - B LEFT - C | GLUTEAL REGION RIGHT - D LEFT - E | DELTOID MUSCLE RIGHT - F LEFT - G | VENTRAL GLUTEAL RIGHT - H LEFT - J | ABDOMINAL RIGHT - K LEFT - L | UPPER ARM RIGHT - R LEFT - S |

| SCHEDULED MEDICATIONS MEDICATION-DOSAGE-FREQUENCY-ROUTE | TIME | DATE | DATE | DATE | DATE | DATE |
|---|---|---|---|---|---|---|
| START 3/5 STOP  Lanoxin 0.25 mg po qd | 10 | | | | | |
| 3/5  Bumex 2mg po qd | 10 | | | | | |
| 3/5  Potassium Cl sol 20 meq tid c̄ juice | 10 / 14 / 18 | | | | | |
| 3/5  Isordil 30mg po q8h | 7 / 15 / 23 | | | | | |
| 3/5  Omnipen-N 1 g IV PB q6h | 6 / 12 / 18 / 24 | | | | | |
| 3/5  MS 2mg IV q3h prn chest pain | | | | | | |
| 3/5  Dalmane 15mg po HS prn sleep | | | | | | |

| PRN MEDICATIONS | | | | SINGLE ORDERS AND PRE-OPS | | |
|---|---|---|---|---|---|---|
| INITIALS | FULL SIGNATURE | TITLE | DATE | MEDICATION-DOSAGE-ROUTE | TIME | INITIALS |
| MI | Michele Iinuma | AN | 3/5 | | | |

| ROOM | PATIENT NAME | | AM | | | PM | |
|---|---|---|---|---|---|---|---|
| 445 | Jones, Mary | M | 1 2 3 4 5 6 7 8 9 10 11 | N | 1 2 3 4 5 6 7 8 9 10 11 | | |

Answer: Page 17

| ALLERGIES | | IV FLUIDS | | LAB | | X-RAY | |
|---|---|---|---|---|---|---|---|
| SULFA | | 3/5 | 500 mL D5W KVO | 3/5 LYTES 3/6 | | DATE | |
| | | | | 3/5 Dig Level 3/6 | | 3/5 Chest XR 3/6 | |

| MEDICATIONS | |
|---|---|
| DATE | |
| 3/5 | Lanoxin 0.25mg po qd |
| 3/5 | Bumex 2mg po qd |
| 3/5 | Potassium (K) 504 20 meq po tid |
| 3/5 | Isordil 30mg po q6h |
| 3/5 | Omnipen-N 1g IVPB q6h |

| TREATMENTS & PROCEDURES | |
|---|---|
| DATE | |
| 3/5 | WEIGH 8AM |
| 3/5 | Call Dr. Lurie if chest pain not relieved by MS (morphine) |

| RESPIRATORY THERAPY | |
|---|---|
| DATE | |

| VITAL SIGNS | DATE | PCMS√s |
|---|---|---|
| DATE | 3/5 q4h | |

| ACTIVITY | |
|---|---|
| 3/5 | MS 2mg IV q3h prn chest pain. |
| 3/5 | Dalmane 15mg po HS prn |

| I/O | S/A | S/G |
|---|---|---|

DIET: 2g Sodium

| ACTIVITY | |
|---|---|
| DATE | |
| 3/5 | Bedrest c̄ BRP |

EMERGENCY NOTIFICATION: Sam Jones 739-0610

SURGERY PROCEDURE

SEX: M (F)   AGE: 69   ADMIT TIME 0900   ADMIT DATE 3/5

CHRONIC MED. PROBLEM

ADM. DIAG. CHF

PHYSICIAN LURIE    CONSULT    NAME: JONES, MARY

HOSP.#372 040865   ROOM # 445

SJ 60265 - REV 11/91

# How To Use *The Physician's Desk Reference* (PDR)

Before administering any medication to a patient the nurse must know the following about each drug.

> The action of the drug
> Indications and classification
> Contraindications
> Adverse reactions to the drug
> Dosage
> Nursing considerations for administering the drug

There are many excellent resources to obtain this information. The one that is usually available on hospitals units is *The Physician's Desk Reference* (PDR). The PDR is a compendium of information that is published by the drug companies. The information can also be found in the package inserts. The PDR is published annually. Hospitals usually replace the PDR annually with a current edition. The nurse must become familiar with using the PDR.

Other resources you will find very helpful are nursing drug handbooks. These books are succinct, contain nursing applications, specific information on how to administer medications and are easy to use. However, they contain fewer drugs than the PDR. The PDR is a compendium of information that is published by the drug companies and contains the same information that appears in package inserts. The PDR is more complete, is research oriented, and contains more drugs than a nursing drug handbook. It is a good idea to use both the PDR and a nursing drug handbook. However, this section is directed at your learning how to use the PDR.

The PDR includes:

| | |
|---|---|
| Section One: | Manufacturers Index (white pages) |
| Section Two:* | Brand and Generic name Index (pink pages) |
| Section Three: | Product Category Index (blue pages) |
| Section Four: | Product Identification Guide (gray pages) |
| Section Five:* | Product Information (white pages) |
| Section Six: | Diagnostic Product Information (green pages) |

*You will primarily be using section two and section five.

## Section One, (white pages) Manufacturers Index

The Manufacturers Index includes each company's address, phone, fax, emergency medical contact, and the products carried. The manufacturers are in alphabetical order. The products are listed in alphabetical order under each manufacturer (mfg). The page numbers to the right of the manufacturer and product indicate the location in which more information may be found. If there are two numbers listed, the first refers to a photograph of the product. If a nurse has a tablet and needs to know the name of the product, this index may help identify the tablet. However, not all products are shown in this section.

Example: Roche Products Inc. 334, 2612

*This page gives information about the product*

page number of photo

## Section Two, (pink pages)  Brand and Generic Name Index

An order for a medication may be written for either the generic name or the trade name.  The generic name is the official name of the drug. This name may reflect the chemical family to which the drug belongs. However, this name is simpler than the chemical name. The brand name is the name the manufacturer chooses to call the product.

The Brand and Generic Name Index includes the products by brand and generic names listed together alphabetically. The generic names are underlined. Brand names are listed under the generic name and again are in alphabetical order. The brand names are followed by the manufacturer's name.

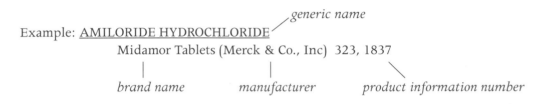

Example: <u>AMILORIDE HYDROCHLORIDE</u>  *generic name*

Midamor Tablets (Merck & Co., Inc)  323, 1837

*brand name*          *manufacturer*          *product information number*

After you find the product in this index, you will use the second number to find product information.

## Section Three, (blue pages)  Product Category Index

The Product Category Index lists all fully described products by prescribing category. The first two pages list a product category quick-reference guide. The product category Index lists categories in alphabetical order with products, manufacturers, and corresponding page numbers. Some examples of drug categories are anti-inflamatory agents, antibiotics—Cephalosporins, cardiovascular agents, and cold preparations.

Example: AIDS Related Complex (ARC) - Prescribing Category

Therapeutic Agents

Bactrim DS Tablets (Roche Laboratories) 324,2614

*product*          *manufacture*          *page number*

## Section Four (gray pages) Product Category Guide

The Product Identification Guide shows actual size photographs in color of tablets and capsules. A variety of other dosages and packages are listed at less than actual size. The products are arranged alphabetically by manufacturer and list the brand name, generic name, and page number for product information.

Example:

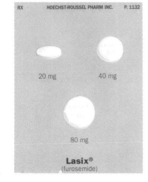

**Note:** *Page numbers will change each year with the new edition of the PDR.*

## Section Five (white pages) Product Information

The Product Information section provides information on nearly 3000 pharmaceuticals. Entries are arranged alphabetically by manufacturer. To look up a specific drug, use the Brand and Generic name index (pink pages) and go to the page number indicated.

Information is given about the products such as descriptions, clinical pharmacology, indications and usage, contraindications, adverse reactions, dosage administration and other information. It is important to remember that the information concerning adverse reactions is very general and various individuals can range from no reactions to serious reactions.

As discussed before, the nurse must know the following about each medication before giving it to the patient. You will find this information in the PDR under the following headings:

| | |
|---|---|
| The action of the drug | Clinical pharmacology |
| Indications | Indications and Usage |
| Contraindications | Contraindications |
| Adverse reactions to the drug | Adverse reactions |
| Dosage | Dosage and Administration |
| What are the nursing considerations for administering the drug | Precautions and Dosage and Administration |

Example: To find information on the drug Lanoxin. Look in the Brand and Generic index (pink pages). Go to the page number indicated which will be the Product Information (white pages).

## Section Six (green pages) Diagnostic Product Information

This section gives usage guidelines for a variety of common diagnostic agents and is arranged alphabetically by manufacturer.

38. Look up Lanoxin 0.25 mg  po qd tablets in the PDR and a nursing drug handbook.

    a. How would you look for Lanoxin in the PDR?

    b. Where would you find information about Lanoxin?

    c. In which section would a photograph of a tablet be found?

    d. Is Lanoxin a generic name or brand name?

    e. What is the action of Lanoxin?

    f. What are the indications for Lanoxin?

    g. What are the contraindications for administering Lanoxin?

    h. What are some of the adverse reactions to Lanoxin?

    i Will the adverse reactions listed be seen in all patients?

    j. What is the usual maintenance dose of Lanoxin?

    k. What are the nursing considerations for administering Lanoxin?

39. Look up Bumex 2 mg  po qd in the PDR and a nursing drug handbook.

    a. Is Bumex the brand name or generic name of the drug?

    b. What is the action of Bumex?

    c. What are the indications for Bumex?

    d. What are the contraindications for administering Bumex?

    e. What are some of the adverse reactions to Bumex?

    f. What is the usual dose of Bumex?

    g. What are the nursing considerations for administering Bumex?

40. Look up potassium chloride sol 20 mEq po tid in the PDR and a nursing drug handbook.

    a. Is potassium chloride the brand name or generic name for the drug?

    b. What is the action of potassium chloride?

    c. What are the indications for potassium chloride?

    d. What are the contraindications for administering potassium chloride?

    e. What are some of the adverse reactions to potassium chloride?

    f. What is the usual dose of potassium chloride?

    g. What are the nursing considerations for administering potassium chloride?

41. Look up morphine sulfate 3-5 mg IV push prn for chest pain in the PDR and a  nursing drug handbook.

    a.  Is morphine sulfate the brand name or the generic name for the drug?

    b.  What is the action of morphine sulfate?

    c.  What are the indications for morphine sulfate?

    d.  What are the contraindications for administering morphine sulfate?

    e.  What are some of the adverse reactions to morphine sulfate?

    f.  What is the usual dose of morphine sulfate?

    g.  What are the nursing considerations for administering morphine sulfate?

Answers: Chapter 1, 38 a-k

38 a. The brand & generic name index.

b. Look up second number in brand & generic index (pink pages) which would send you to the product information section (white pages).

c. Use the first number on the brand & generic name index then turn to the Product Category Guide.

d. Brand.

e. An increase in the force and velocity of myocardial systolic contraction (positive inotropic action) and a slowing of heart rate (negative chronotropic effect) and a decreased conduction through the AV node. This leads to better circulation and reduced swelling of the hands and ankles in patients with heart failure.

f. heart failure, atrial fibrillation, atrial flutter and paroxysmal atrial tachycardia.

g. digitalis toxicity, ventricular fibrillation, and ventricular tachycardia. h. fatigue, generalized muscle weakness, agitation, hallucinations, yellow green halo around field of vision, anorexia, nausea, vomiting, diarrhea i. No j. 0.25 mg per day. k. Oral or IV route most desirable because IM injection is extremely painful. Before giving, take the apical pulse for 1 full minute - if less than 60 hold dose and notify the physician, check potassium level - low potassium level can increase the risk of digitalis toxicity, check serum levels of digoxin, therapeutic range is 0.5 - 2 ng/mL IV Lanoxin should be given over 5 minutes.

Answers: Chapter 1, 39 a-g

39 a. Bumex is the brand name - bumetanide is the generic name.  b. Bumex is a loop diuretic with rapid onset and short duration that inhibits sodium and chloride reabsorption in the ascending portion of the loop of Henle. Loop diuretics are given to help reduce the amount of water in the body. They work by acting on the kidneys to increase the flow of urine.  c. Treatment of edema associated with congestive heart failure, hepatic disease and renal disease.  d. anuria, hepatic coma, severe electrolyte depletion until corrected. Contraindicated for any patient who is hypersensitive to the drug.  e. Muscle cramps, dizziness, headache, volume and electrolyte depletion, dehydration, orthostatic hypotension, and rash.  f. The usual is 0.5-2mg once a day. May be given po, IV or IM. If diuretic response is not adequate a second and third dose may be given in 2-3 hour intervals. Maximum dose is 10 mg/day.  g. Bumex should be given in the morning to prevent the increase of urination from affecting sleep. If a second dose is needed, it should be given before 6 PM. (This does not apply in critical care situations). Monitor intake & output, daily weight, serum electrolytes especially potassium - can lead to potassium loss and may need to be given in conjunction with a potassium supplement. Bumex can lead to water and electrolyte depletion - monitor pulse rate and blood pressure during diuresis. When given intravenously, give over 1-2 minutes.

Answers; Chapter 1, 40 a-g

40 a. generic.

b. Replaces and maintains serum potassium level.

c. Potassium replacement - especially for patients who are on loop diuretics that may increase the loss of potassium in the urine. This is determined by the serum potassium. Normal serum potassium 3.5-5mEq per liter less than 3.5 indicates a need for potassium replacement.

d. Contraindications are hyperkalemia, oliguria, or anuria or severe renal impairment.

e. hyperkalemia, GI ulcerations and GI hemorrhage, nausea, vomiting, abdominal pain, oliguria, EKG changes such as widened QRS complex, prolonged PR interval, tall tented T waves, and ST segment depression.

f. Antihypokalemic dosage is 15-25 mEq two to four times per day, the dosage being adjusted as needed and tolerated.

g. Monitor serum potassium levels, monitor intake and output, give with or after meals on a full stomach with a full glass of water or juice to lessen gastrointestinal distress, solid tablet dosage forms should not be used in patients with delayed gastric emptying, esophageal compression, or intestinal stricture. The use of potassium tablets in such conditions increases the possibility of tissue destruction by high, local concentrations of potassium released by the tablet. Potassium sol is the preferred choice in these situations.

Answers: Chapter 1, 41 a-g

41 a. morphine sulfate is the generic name for the drug.

b. morphine sulfate is an opiate analgesic. The principle actions of morphine are analgesia-pain relief, and sedation. The precise mechanism of action is unknown. Specific CNS opiate receptors and endogenous compounds with morphine-like activity have been identified throughout the brain and spinal cord and are likely to play a role in the expression of analgesic effect.

c. Used for the relief of moderate to severe pain. Morphine is the drug of choice to relieve pain due to acute myocardial infarction.

d. Contraindicated in patients who are hypersensitive to this drug or other opiates.

e. Respiratory depression, sedation, somnolence, clouded sensorium, euphoria, dizziness, hypotension, bradycardia, urinary retention, and physical dependence or addiction.  f. Usual intravenous dosage is 2.5 to 15 mg.

g. Dilute the Morphine 10 mg/ml in 9 ml of sterile water for a total volume of 10 ml. This provides a concentration of 1 mg/ml. Titrate the dose according to patient response. Give over 2-3 minutes. Morphine can cause respiratory depression - monitor vital signs frequently especially respirations. Have Narcan on hand to reverse the effects of Morphine should respiratory depression or excessive sedation become a problem. The intravenous push route of morphine should only be used in situations where the patient can be closely monitored such as the Emergency Room, Intensive Care Unit, or the Recovery Room. Morphine is a controlled substance since its use can become addictive. Constipation may be a problem with continued use.

# Reading Drug Labels

Drug labels must be read carefully. Medications are packaged in containers with a label that gives information on the contents and directions for its administration. The unit dose label is the most common type of packaging found in the hospital setting. Unit dosage is each drug packaged and labeled in a single unit. For example, each tablet or capsule is packaged in a separate wrapper. Such packaging ensures complete identification of the drug until it is given. The drug should remain sealed in its wrapper until it is given to the patient. Multiple dose containers may also be encountered.

The brand or trade name is the commercial name given the drug by the pharmaceutical company. A drug can have many brand names, each given by a different drug company. The generic name is the official name of the drug as listed in the United States Pharmacopeia (USP) and the National Formulary (NF). Each drug has only one official generic name.

What to look for on the drug label

- Drug name trade name—generic name or both

- Dosage strength per unit such as per mL, per tablet, or capsule

- The route of administration - not always indicated on the label

- Total amount per vial or bottle

- Company name that manufactured the drug

- Expiration date of the drug

- Directions for reconstitution or storage of the drug

*Sample Problem*

**Generic name:** nifedipine
Since only one name is shown on this label, it is the generic name. If this drug was ordered with the trade name, Procardia, and filled by the pharmacist with nifedipine, the nurse would have to look up the drug to be certain it is the same drug.
**Dosage per capsule:** 10 mg
**Route:** oral

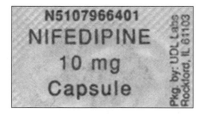

**Dosage per unit measure**: 300 mg /2mL
**Trade name**: Tagamet
**Generic name**: cimetidine HCL
**Route**: injection
**Company name**: Smith Kline Beechham
**Total dose per vial**: 8 mL.
Do not confuse the total amount in the vial with the dosage per unit measure. 300 mg/2mL would be used for the drug calculation.

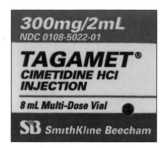

**Total amount per vial**: 500 mg
**Trade name**: Ancef
**Generic name**: cefazolin
**Route**: IM or IV
**Dosage strength:** if mixed for IM
use 225 mg/mL
**Instructions:** add 2 mL of sterile water and shake well. May store at room temperature for 24 hours or refrigerated for 10 days.
**Company name**: SmithKline Beecham

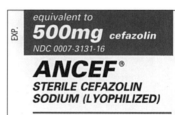

**Generic name**: potassium chloride
**Dosage per unit measure**: 20mEq per 15 mL
**Route**: oral solution
**USP**: abbreviation for United States Pharmacopeia. It is one of the agencies that provides the national official listing of drugs.
**Company name**: Roxane Laboratories
Instructions: must be diluted in water or juice before administering.

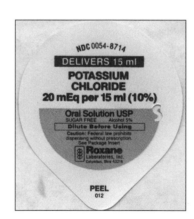

**Reading Drug Labels**

For each of the problems below fill in the blanks

42. a.  Trade name      _____

    b.  Generic name      _____

    c.  Dosage per unit      _____

    d.  Total mL per bottle      _____

    e.  Route      _____

    f.  Company      _____

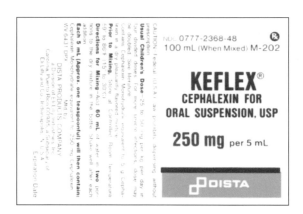

43. a.  Generic name      _____

    b.  Dosage per unit      _____

    c.  Route      _____

    d.  Company      _____

    e.  Warning      _____

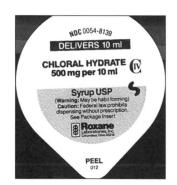

44. a.  Trade name      _____

    b.  Generic name      _____

    c.  Dosage per unit      _____

    d.  Total mL per bottle      _____

    e.  Route      _____

    f.  Company      _____

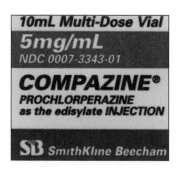

45. a. Trade name      _____

     b. Generic name      _____

     c. Dosage per unit      _____

     d. Number tablets/
        container      _____

     e. Route      _____

     f. Company      _____

N 0071-0569-24

**Nitrostat®**
(Nitroglycerin
Tablets, USP)

**0.3 mg (1/200 gr)**

Caution—Federal law prohibits
dispensing without prescription.

100 SUBLINGUAL TABLETS

Ⓟ **PARKE-DAVIS**
People Who Care

46. a. Trade name      _____

     b. Generic name      _____

     c. Dosage per vial      _____

     d. Route      _____

     e. Company      _____

     f. Directions      _____

     g. Information needed on
        label after mixing      _____

                _____

**Cefizox®**
(sterile ceftizoxime sodium)

FUJISAWA

equivalent to
**1 gram**
ceftizoxime

For Intravenous
Admixture

Single-Dose
Piggyback Vial

NDC 0469-7252-01      725201

Each vial contains: Ceftizoxime sodium equivalent to 1 gram of
ceftizoxime. The sodium content is 60 mg (2.6 mEq) per gram of
ceftizoxime activity.

Primarily for institutional use.

**Usual Dosage:** See Package Insert.

Reconstitution: Add 50 to 100 mL of Sodium Chloride Injection or
other intravenous solution listed in package insert. Shake well.
Administer as single dose with primary intravenous fluids.

This reconstituted solution of Cefizox® is stable 24 hours at room
temperature or 96 hours if refrigerated (5°C).

**CAUTION:** Federal law prohibits dispensing without prescription.

Product of Japan
Manufactured for Fujisawa USA, Inc., Deerfield, IL 60015 by Smith Kline Beecham,
Philadephia, PA 19101      693831B/B94

Prepared By / Date Prepared / Time / Patient

**Cefizox® equivalent to
1 gram ceftizoxime**

# How Drugs Are Supplied

### Tablets, Capsules, Caplets

The majority of drugs given by mouth come in tablet, capsule, or caplet form for the adult patient. They may not be broken in half unless scored. Oral drugs are ordered in milligrams, grams, grains, or units. When there is more than one strength of a drug, it is best to select the strength so the fewest number of pills are given. Double check with a licensed person whenever more than three tablets are ordered. It is rare that more than three tablets are given. If so, there may be an error in transcribing, calculating or prescribing. Use Clean technique.

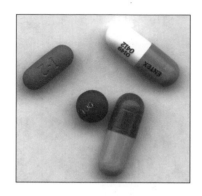

### Scored Tablets

These tablets are scored so they can easily be broken to give half the dosage. Use Clean technique.

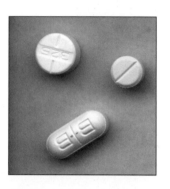

### Long Acting or Sustained Release Tablets

Patient compliance increases when the drug is prescribed once or twice a day rather than three or four times a day. Many drugs come in a longer acting form. Look for the abbreviations SA, LA or XL. This means that all of the drug is not released immediately but gradually from 12-24 hours. Be alert to this when reading labels and transcribing orders. Do not give 60 mg of immediate release Procardia when the long acting form is what was ordered. These tablets may not be crushed, chewed or broken. Use Clean technique.

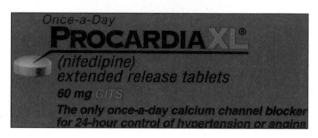

Once-a-Day
**PROCARDIA XL®**
(nifedipine)
extended release tablets
**60 mg** GITS
The only once-a-day calcium channel blocker for 24-hour control of hypertension or angina

| LABELS WHICH INDICATE NOT TO BE CHEWED, CRUSHED OR BROKEN | SYMBOLS FOR SUSTAINED RELEASE |
|---|---|
| | Dur |
| | SR |
| Bid as in Theobid | CR |
| (E.C.) Enteric Coated | SA |
| Spansules | Contin |
| Extentabs | LA |
| Extencaps | LX |

## Sublingual Tablets

Sublingual tablets are placed under the tongue where they are absorbed very rapidly. Sublingual may be abbreviated SL on the label. Use Clean technique.

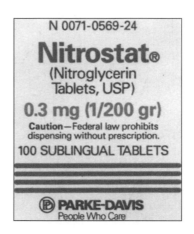

## Liquid Medication—Suspensions, Syrup, Oral Solution and Elixirs

Many drugs also come in liquid form and are used for children and adults who cannot swallow tablets or capsules. They are also easier to pass through a nasogastric tube or gastrostomy tube. Liquid medications are measured in teaspoons or milliliters. Use Clean technique.

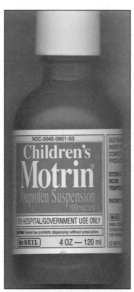

## Rectal Suppositories

Drugs may be given via the rectum and come in the form of a suppository. They are very useful when the patient is nauseated and can not take the oral form of the drug. Compazine suppositories are frequently given for nausea. Many drugs may not be given this route. Use Clean technique and wear gloves.

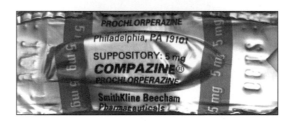

## Vaginal Suppositories and Creams

A few drugs may be given vaginally and are available in creams or suppositories. Estrace is a vaginal cream usually administered at bedtime. Use Clean technique and wear gloves.

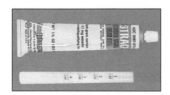

## Medications for the Eye

Eye drops or ointments must be clearly labeled for the eye. Look for ophthalmic solution or ointment on the label. Only ophthalmic preparations of the drug may be used in the eyes. Severe damage to the eye could occur if some other preparation were used. Be especially careful with ear drops so as not to confuse them with eye drops. Double check the order to determine if it is the right eye (OD), left eye (OS), or both eyes (OU). Use steile technique. To maintain sterility of container, do not touch the eye lid when administering the drops.

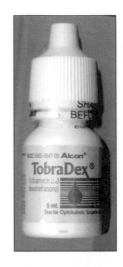

## Medications for the Ear

Look for otic on the label which indicates the preparation is for the ear. Again, double check the order to determine if its for the right ear, left ear, or both ears. The abbreviation for ear is AU. Otic medications are prescribed in drops. The usual dosage of Cortisporin is 4 drops 3 or 4 times per day. Use clean technique.

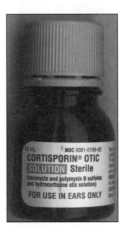

## Transdermal Drug Patches

Drugs are also administered through the skin in the form of pastes or patches. The drug is absorbed slowly through the skin as it leeches out of a matrix or is released through a microporous membrane. The Transderm-Nitro shown in the picture is changed every 24 hours. Some patches are changed once a week. The patches come in different strengths. Read the label to ascertain the right strength. Check the patch for size and dosage per hour. Look for and remove the old patch before adding a new one. Apply the patch to the torso rather than an extremity.

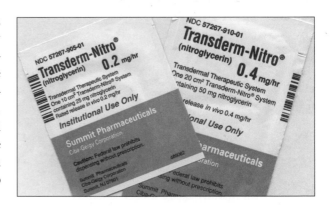

Frequent movement of a patient's arm increases the circulation and will alter the rate of absorption of the drug. Apply at the same time each day and write the day and time applied on the patch.

Never apply heat to the patched area. Heat increases the rate of absorption. This could result in a dangerous overdosage. Use clean technique.

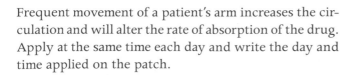

## Metered Inhalers

Inhalers give a measured or metered dose per "puff" on inhalation to the respiratory system. The usual dose of Ventolin is 2 puffs every 4-6 hours as needed. With the Ventolin inhaler, each puff delivers about 90 mg of Ventolin (albuterol) to the respiratory system. Correct use of an inhaler requires the patient to fully exhale, time the "puff" with inhalation and hold the breath as long as possible after inhalation. Observe patients while they are using the inhaler to be sure it is being operated correctly. The right dosage occurs when the inhaler is used properly with the prescribed number of inhalations. The patients should notify their doctor if they do not get relief with the prescribed dosage.

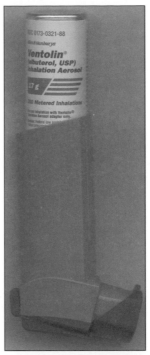

## Parenteral Drugs

Injectable drugs may be supplied in an ampule. An ampule is a single dose container. The neck of the ampule is scored and can be easily broken by snapping the top of the ampule into a gauze as shown. Read the label and package insert for the route the drug may be given. Many injectables may be given IV, IM, or SQ. Some may be given only by one route. Use sterile technique.

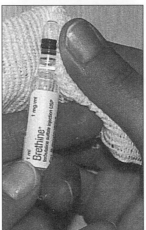

## Drawing Medication From an Ampule

The drug can be drawn into a syringe by holding the ampule as shown. Draw the medication into the syringe that is prescribed and discard the portion that is not needed. Use sterile technique.

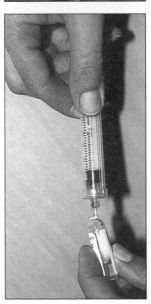

## Vials-Parenteral Drugs

Many injectable drugs are supplied in vials. Vials may be of single or multiple dose size. Pay close attention to the Versed vial label which indicates the route. It can be used for IM or IV use. It is not for subcutaneous (SQ) use. Vials have a resealable rubber diaphragm in the top. Use sterile technique.

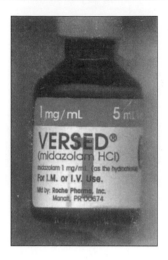

To withdraw the drug, the needle is inserted into the diaphragm. The diaphragm must be cleansed with an antiseptic before inserting the needle. If you are withdrawing 2 mL of Versed, you would first inject 2 mL of air into the vial and then invert the vial as shown in the picture. The air prevents a vacuum from forming after the drug is withdrawn. Use sterile technique.

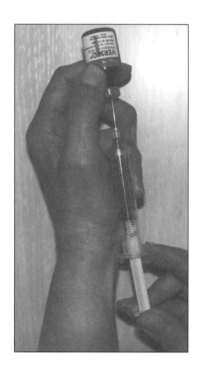

## Single Dosage Pre-filled Tubex

Pharmaceutical companies prepare many drugs in single dosage, pre-filled tubex or syringes. The Toradol tubex is slipped into a cartridge to be administered. The usual dosage of Toradol is 30 mg, so 1 mL would be given (all of the solution). If only 15 mg of Toradol was ordered, 0.5 mL of solution would be given and 0.5 mL discarded. Use sterile technique.

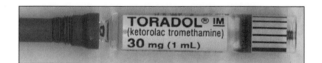

Drugs can be given by Nasal Spray. This container has 120 doses of 50 mcg per spray. The usual dosage is one spray daily in each nostril. Have the patient tilt their head forward slightly and while holding one nostril, press down to administer the spray, during inhalation.

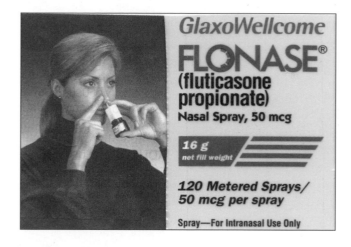

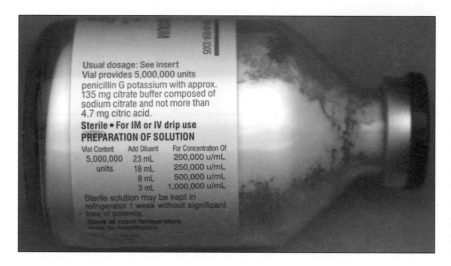

**Penicillin Pwd + 8 mL water = 10 mL**

It might be asked, why not just add 10 mL of sterile saline to the vial. The powdered penicillin adds to the total amount, therefore, if you added 10 mL of solution, the total would equal 12 mL instead of 10 mL. The manufacturer has figured exactly how much is needed for four different concentrations of penicillin in solution. When you mix penicillin or any other drug, write the date, time, amount of the drug per mL, and your name on the label.

## Reconstitution of Parenteral Drugs

Parental drugs may be packaged in powdered form to increase the shelf life of the drug. In dried powdered form the drug will remain good until the expiration date on the vial. After the drug is mixed with a solution, it loses its potency within a short period of time. It may only remain potent for a day at room temperature or a few days if refrigerated. This information will be specified on either the drug label or package insert.

Penicillin G can be reconstituted four different ways. Read instructions on the label. If you want 500,000 units per mL, you would add 8 mL of sterile saline to the vial.

# Equipment Utilized for Drug Administration

### 3 mL or 3 cc Syringe

The 3 mL syringe is the most commonly used syringe for intramuscular (IM) injections. It is used with a 1 to 1.5 inch needle. Intramuscular means that the drug is deposited into the muscle, below the subcutaneous layer. This is why a longer needle is used. The length of the needle is determined by the site and how much subcutaneous tissue is present. Absorption is more rapid from the intramuscular site than the subcutaneous tissue. The IM route is used for drugs that are more irritating and require a more rapid onset. Intramuscular medications should not be given in amounts greater than 3 mL. The muscle can not readily absorb more than 3 mL of solution. The 3 mL syringe measures accurately to one-tenth of a mL. Each 1 mL is calibrated with 10 lines. Each calibration line equals 1/10 of a mL.

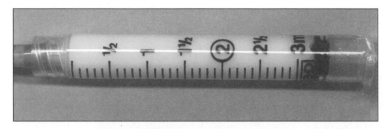

This syringe has measured 0.7 mL of a drug. Count 7 lines. See the arrow.

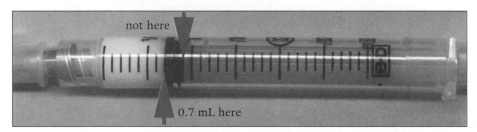

### Tuberculin Syringe

The tuberculin syringe is used mainly for intradermal or subcutaneous injections. They are supplied with a ½ inch or 5/8 inch needle, which is the appropriate length for these injections. **Intradermal means** the medication is deposited into the dermal layers of the skin until a small wheal is produced. This type of injection is done for the purpose of skin testing. The TB (tuberculin) skin test is one of the most common intradermal tests. When the tuberculin syringe is used for **subcutaneous injections, absorption is slower, but the effects last longer.** SusPhrine for asthmatic patients is an example of a drug that is given subcutaneously because of its slower rate of absorption. If SusPhrine was given IM, it could cause cardiac arrhythmia. The subcutaneous tissue is over the muscle and just under the skin. To keep from injecting the medication into the muscle, this shorter 1/2 or 5/8 inch needle is used. The skin and subcutaneous tissue is pinched for the injection and a 45 degree angle is used. If the tuberculin syringe is used to give an intramuscular injection, the needle must be changed to at least 1 inch. Notice with the tuberculin syringe that 1 mL is calibrated with **10 large lines measuring 1/10 mL.** In between each 1/10 mL markings are smaller lines. **Each smaller line measures 1/100 of a mL.** To measure 0.25 mL, count 5 lines past the 0.2 mL marker. See the arrow. Usually the volume of medication given subcutaneously is limited to 1 mL.

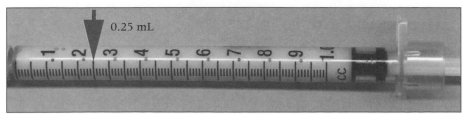

### U-100 Insulin Syringe

Insulin is also given subcutaneously because of its slower and longer rate of absorption. There are special syringes just for the purpose of measuring insulin. U-100 insulin syringes are supplied with a ½ inch and 5/8 inch needles for subcutaneous injection of insulin. It is also made with a very small, 27 gauge needle, and holds up to 100 units of insulin. The syringe is marked at the 10, 20, 30, 40 units etc. In between each 10 units are 4 lines. Each line measures **2 units** of insulin. To measure 58 units, count 4 lines past the 50 unit marker. See the arrow.

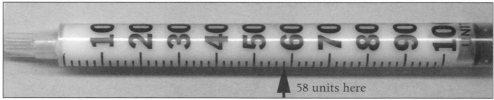

58 units here

### U-100 Low Dose Insulin Syringe

This syringe is also for U-100 insulin. It is designed for smaller doses of insulin. It can only measure up to 50 units of insulin. Notice that each calibration measures **1 unit** of insulin. It is especially useful for diabetics and children, where very accurate measurement is important. To measure 7 units of insulin, count seven lines. See the arrow.

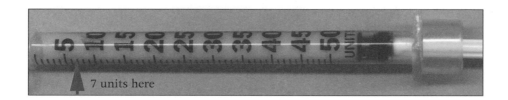

7 units here

**Note:** *Insulin syringes are used only for insulin administration.*

### The Ounce Cup

Oral medications which come in liquid suspensions or elixirs are measured in an ounce cup. Liquid medications are measured in teaspoons, milliliters, tablespoons, drams and ounces. The ounce cup has the various measurements on the side of the cup. Different sides of the cup have different measurements. An ounce cup measures to 1 tsp or 1 dram. Hold the once cup at eye level and read from the bottom of the meniscus.

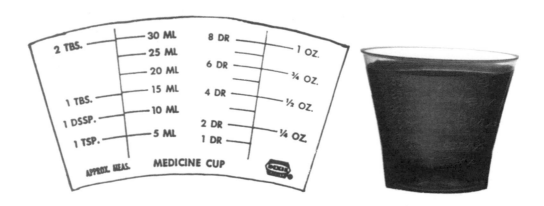

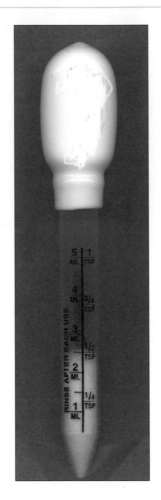

## Calibrated Dropper

Liquid drugs may be measured by a calibrated dropper. Several liquid drugs are supplied by the pharmaceutical company with the calibrated dropper.

## The infusion Pump

Accurate delivery of intravenous drugs is best accomplished by using an infusion pump. Infusion pumps use special tubing which is inserted into a controller device inside the machine. On the front panel the desired number of mL/h is set by the R.N. The infusion rate range is from 1 - 999 mL/h. If the infusion pump cannot maintain the set rate of m/h, it will alarm. Intravenous drug dosages may be ordered per hour, per minute, and per kilogram per minute. The R.N. must determine the number of **mL/h which will deliver the correct drug dosage.** The nurse calculates the number of mL/h necessary to deliver the dosage ordered, and then sets the machine to deliver that designated number of mL/h.

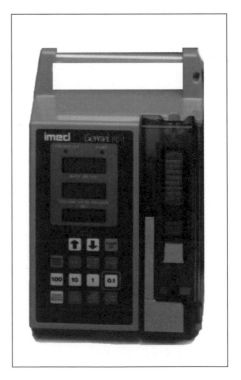

## IV Peripheral Catheters

The intravenous route for drug administration in many cases is replacing IM injections. This route has the advantage of rapid and precise absorption. It also saves the patient from repeated injections. The catheter is inserted in any peripheral vein with the needle inside the plastic catheter. After the vein is accessed, the needle is removed and the plastic catheter remains in the vein.

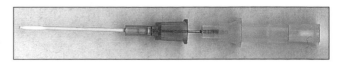

## Saline or Heparin Lock (HL)

The IV peripheral catheter can be left as a saline lock for intermittent IV drug administration for example, an antibiotic that is prescribed q8h. The saline lock is flushed with saline or heparin following the antibiotic to keep the catheter open. This allows the patient increased mobility between drug doses. Saline or Heparin locks are also used for many hospital inpatients who might need intravenous access for administration of emergency drugs. In this case its a prophylactic measure during the time they are unstable.

saline lock port

plastic catheter

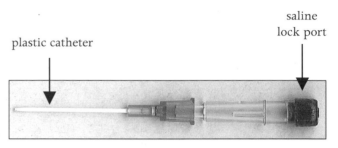

## IV Piggyback (IV PB)

An IV piggyback is a secondary line piggyback to a primary infusion. See the picture. The primary line hangs below the secondary line. When the secondary line is finished, the primary infusion continues to run again. The IV does not run dry with this system.

secondary piggyback

primary line

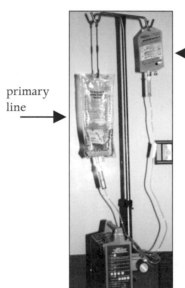

## Protection Against Bloodborne Pathogens

The National Institute for Occupational Safety and Health Administration (OSHA), and the Centers for Disease Control and Prevention (CDC) require Universal Precautions, Proper Sharps Disposal, and Needleless IV Systems. Universal Precautions requires wearing gloves for any procedure, with any patient, which may result in exposure to blood or bodily fluids. All sharps must be disposed into a rigid, puncture resistant, leak proof container, specifically designated for sharps. Needleless IV Systems include IV access ports that do not use needles.

IVAC Corporations Needleless System.

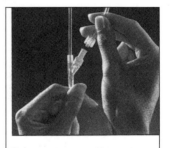

Connect a secondary set or syringe using a luer-lock

---

**NEEDLE STICK PREVENTION**

1. Needles are not to be used in IV tubing whether you are giving an IV push drug or connecting an IV PB to a "Y" site.
2. Never recap a needle after use.
3. Always immediately dispose of needles in the appropriate sharps container.

## IV Tubing with access ports that do not require a needle.

IV PB and IV pushes can be connected without the use of a needle. The medication will need to be drawn up with a sterile needle and then detached just before the drug is given. This helps to prevent needle sticks with contaminated needles.

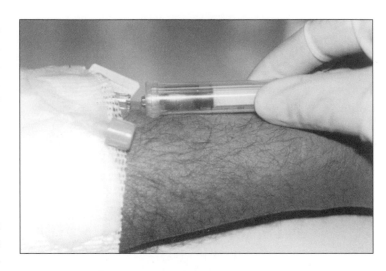

## IV Push

Some drugs may be given directly by IV push and do not need to be diluted. Drugs can be given IV push by RNs who have been specially trained in this practice. Hospitals have protocols that state which drugs may be given IV push, where they may be given IV push, and who may give an IV push.

## Syringe Infusion Pumps

The antibiotic cefazolin 1 g is diluted by the pharmacist with 0.45 NS for a total amount of 30 mL in a syringe. The cefazolin is placed in the syringe infusion pump and the pump is set to infuse the drug over 30 minutes. The cefazolin line is connected to the primary IV. Syringe infusion pumps are becoming more popular to reduce costs. The extra bag of diluent for the piggyback is eliminated.

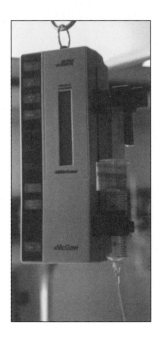

## Multilumen Catheters

Multilumen catheters are used when patients are on numerous drugs and IV fluids that may be incompatible when run in the same line. This catheter is inserted in a central vein and has three individual ports.

three ports
for IV access

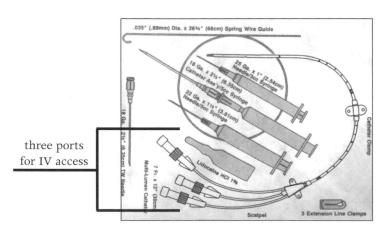

Read the measurement on the 3 mL syringes where the arrow points.

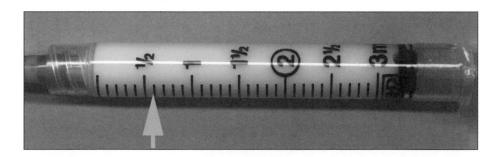

47._____

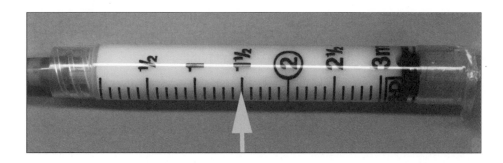

48._____

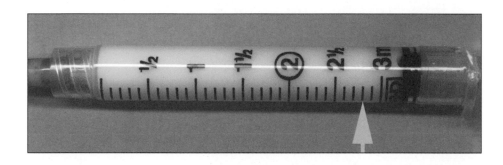

49._____

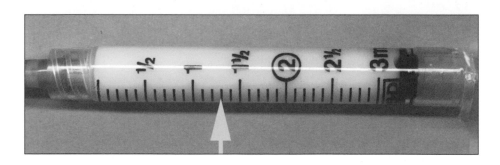

50._____

## Tuberculin Syringes

Read the measurement on each tuberculin syringe where the arrow points

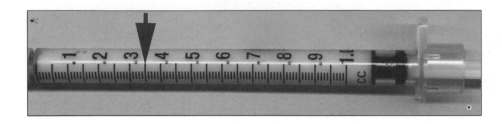

51._____

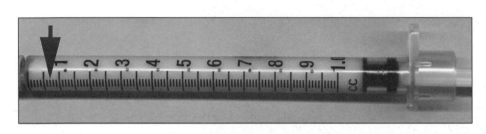

52._____

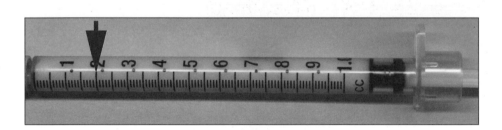

53._____

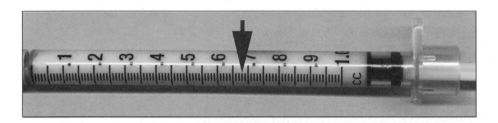

54._____

**Insulin Syringes**

Read the measurement on each insulin syringe where the arrow points

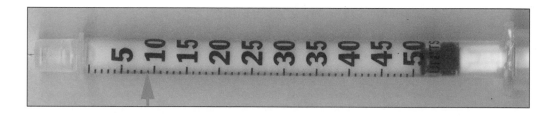

55._____

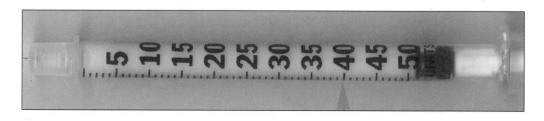

56._____

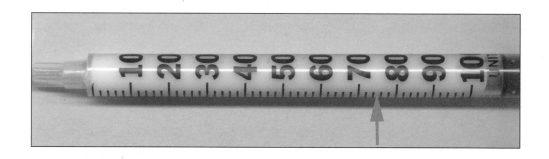

57._____

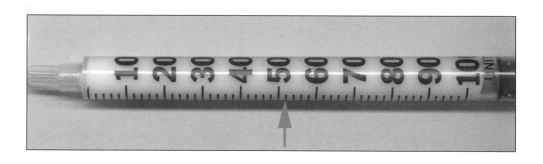

58._____

Answers: Chapter 1, 47-58

| | | | |
|---|---|---|---|
| 47. 0.6 mL | 50. 1.3 mLs | 53. 0.68 mL | 56. 40 units |
| 48. 1.5 mLs | 51. 0.35 mL | 54. 0.2 mL | 57. 75 units |
| 49. 2.8 mLs | 52. 0.07 mL | 55. 9 units | 58. 52 units |

# Summary of Drug Administration

1. Have a physician's order for all drugs given. Check all drugs on the MAR with the Kardex or physician's order sheet at the beginning of each shift.

2. Question any orders or handwriting that is unclear.

3. Calculate correct dosage to prepare the drug.

4. Check for allergies to drugs.

5. Select drugs for the appropriate time. All doses of medication should be administered at scheduled times unless there is a problem to be resolved.

6. If the drug is missing from the patient's cubicle, do not borrow a drug from another patient's cubicle. Contact the pharmacist about the missing drug. There may be a reason it was not filled such as contraindications, allergies or incompatibilities.

7. Wash hands before preparing drugs and before administering drugs to each patient.

8. Read the label three times.

9. Make sure you have the right route for the drug.

10. Determine the specifics of how to administer each drug. Example: potassium solutions must be diluted in water or juice.

11. Check the expiration date on the package of each drug.

12. Only administer drugs you have prepared (except for those prepared by the pharmacist). Drugs should not be removed from their package until just before they are administered.

13. Do not crush capsules, enteric coated tablets and long acting drugs.

14. Check to be sure the patient is not NPO (nothing by mouth) before administering oral medications.

15. Know the action, correct dosage range, adverse reactions, and contraindications before administering any drug.

16. Be aware of nursing considerations or necessary assessments prior to giving a drug. For example, obtain an apical pulse before administering digoxin.

17. Identify the patient by looking at the arm band before administering any medication.

18. Assist the patient in taking the medication.

19. If the patient refuses any medication, recheck the order. If the patient still refuses, chart the reason it was refused and notify the doctor.

20. Observe the patient taking the medication. Do not leave medications at the bedside.

21. Always chart each drug after it is administered, not before.

22. Before giving prn medications, check to see the last time the medication was given to be sure it is not too soon for the next dose.

23. Observe the patient and chart expected outcomes of the drug.

24. Observe the patient for any adverse reactions and report it to the physician.

**This is a summary of general guidelines for safe drug administration. Read the policy and procedures where you work. There may be additional guidelines specific to each area of practice.**

# 2

# Chapter Two

# Ratio
## and
# Proportion

# Ratio and Proportion

## Introduction

Ratio proportion is an effective way to solve and check dosage problems. Although many problems can be calculated mentally, it is a good idea to double check using ratio proportion. Drug calculation problems can be done by using the ratio proportion method of solving for X. Sample and Practice problems for oral and injectable drugs are included in this chapter. Look at the definitions for ratio, proportion and X.

---

### Definitions

**Ratio** expresses the relationship of one quantity to another. It is also a fraction.

Example: 1 is to 3 or 1: 3, or $\dfrac{1}{3}$

**Proportion** shows the relationship between two ratios that are equal.
Example:

$$\frac{1}{3} = \frac{3}{9} \qquad\qquad \frac{1}{3} = \frac{3}{9}$$

$$3 \times 3 = 9 \qquad\qquad 1 \times 9 = 9$$

Since the cross products are equal, the two ratios do form a proportion.

**X** is the unknown number. In any proportion, if you have three out of four numbers, you can calculate the fourth or unknown number.

---

With the above ratio $\dfrac{1}{3} = \dfrac{3}{9}$ let us assume that you do not have one of the numbers. It would then be called X or the unknown number.

$$\frac{3}{X} = \frac{1}{3}$$

X is the unknown

To solve for X, the unknown number can be found by cross-multiplying the denominator on the left with the numerator on the right, and the denominator on the right with the numerator on the left and then dividing the equation by the number in front of the X.

$$\frac{3}{X} = \frac{1}{3}$$

$$1 \times X = 3 \times 3$$

$$1 X = 9$$

$$X = 9$$

■ In summary, the unknown number is 9. In most drug calculation problems, three out of four numbers are available, and the fourth can be calculated by using the ratio proportion method.

# Ratio

A ratio is the correspondence between numbers of two sets.

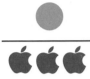

The ratio of oranges to apples is 1 orange to 3 apples, or 1 : 3 or $\frac{1}{3}$

## Proportion
A proportion is a statement of equality between two ratios.

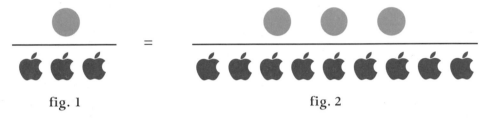

fig. 1                                        fig. 2

The ratio of oranges to apples in figure 1 is proportional to the ratio of oranges to apples in figure 2.

## Ratio Proportion for Drug Calculation
The proportion method works well to solve calculation problems. One type of proportion commonly used is to compare milligrams to milliliters. In figure 3, there are 100 milligrams in 1 milliliter of solution. The question is, what part of 1 milliliter of solution contains 35 milligrams.

| Available from pharmacy demerol 100 mg in 1 mL | | Doctor's Order to Give demerol 35 mg | |
|---|---|---|---|
| numerator = mg | 100 mg | 35 mg | numerator = mg |
| denominator = mL | 1 mL | X mL | denominator = mL |
| | fig. 3 | fig. 4 | |

$$\frac{100 \text{ mg}}{1 \text{ mL}} = \frac{35 \text{ mg}}{X \text{ mL}}$$

Figures 3 and 4 illustrate two ratios which are equal but one number, X, is unknown. To arrange a proportion properly, like units must be placed on the top and like units on the bottom. Notice in figures 3 and 4, mg occurs in both numerators and mL occurs in both denominators. In figures 1 and 2, oranges occur in both numerators and apples occur in both denominators.

**Note:** *Apples and oranges cannot be mixed.*

# Method: Ratio Proportion
# Oral Tablets or Capsules

The following sample problem of Lanoxin (digoxin) uses ratio proportion to decide how many tablets to give.

1. Determine what you are to give (the doctor's order).
2. Determine what is available from the pharmacy by reading the label.
3. Arrange into a ratio proportion with like units in the numerator and like units in the denominator.
4. Cross-multiply.
5. Divide.

*The physician orders Lanoxin 0.25 mg po qd.*

1. **How many mg of Lanoxin should be given to the patient?**

   Answer: Lanoxin 0.25 mg qd.

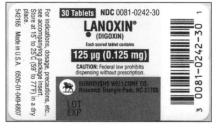

2. **What is available from the pharmacy?**

   Answer: Lanoxin 0.125 mg in one tablet

3. **Arrange ratio proportion. It is helpful to write the known first (0.125 per 1 tablet)**

$$\frac{0.125 \text{ mg}}{1 \text{ tablet}} = \frac{0.25 \text{ mg}}{X \text{ tablets}}$$

4. **Cross-multiply.**

$$\frac{0.125 \text{ mg}}{1 \text{ tablet}} = \frac{0.25 \text{ mg}}{X \text{ tablets}} \qquad \frac{0.125 \text{ mg}}{1 \text{ tablet}} = \frac{0.25 \text{ mg}}{X \text{ tablets}}$$

$$0.125 \text{ X} = 0.25$$

5. **Divide.**

$$\frac{0.125X}{0.125} = \frac{0.25}{0.125}$$

$$X = 2$$

**In summary, to give 0.25 mg to the patient, 2 tablets should be given. Two tablets = 0.25 mg.**

# Method: Formula (Alternate method to ratio proportion) Oral Medications in Liquid Form

*The physician orders Augmentin (amoxicillin) 400 mg po q8h.*

**Formula:**

$$\frac{\text{Desired dose}}{\text{Dose on hand}} \times \text{Quantity} = \text{Amount of drug} \qquad \frac{D}{H} \times Q = A$$

1. Desired dose to be given to patient = Augmentin 400 mg

   D = 400 mg

2. On hand from the pharmacy = Augmentin 200 mg/5 mL

   H = 200 mg

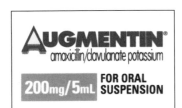

3. Quantity = 5 mL

   Q = 5

4. Calculate the formula

   $$\frac{D}{H} \times Q = A \qquad\qquad \frac{400}{200} \times 5 = 10 \text{ mL}$$

The nurse would pour 10 mL or two teaspoons of Augmentin into an ounce cup.

**Note:** *On the equivalency chart, 1 tsp is equal to 5 mL. If in a different calculation problem your answer will be less than one tsp, change the tsp to 5 mL and work the problem.*

In summary, to give 400 mg of Augmentin to the patient, 10 mL or 2 tsp should be given. 10 mL = 400 mg.

# Method: Ratio Proportion  Oral Liquids

*The physician orders Claritin Syrup (loratadine) 3 mg po qd.*

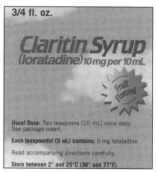

1. **How much Claritin Syrup should be given to the patient?**

   Answer: 3 mg

2. **What is available from the pharmacy?**

   Answer: **Claritin Syrup** 5 mg per tsp

   **Claritin Syrup** 10 mg per 10 mL

**Note:** *On the equivalency chart, 1 tsp is equal to 5 mL. If your answer will be less than one tsp, change the tsp to 5 mL and work the problem. There are no markings on the medicine cup for fractions of a teaspoon.*

   *Change 1 tsp to 5 mL — they are equivalent.

3. **Arrange ratio proportion**

   $$\frac{5 \text{ mg}}{5 \text{ mL}} = \frac{3 \text{ mg}}{X \text{ mL}}$$
   
   or
   
   $$\frac{10 \text{ mg}}{10 \text{ mL}} = \frac{3 \text{ mg}}{X \text{ mL}}$$

4. **Cross-multiply**

   $$\frac{5 \text{ mg}}{5 \text{ mL}} = \frac{3 \text{ mg}}{X \text{ mL}} \qquad \frac{5 \text{ mg}}{5 \text{ mL}} = \frac{3 \text{ mg}}{X \text{ mL}}$$
   
   or
   
   $$\frac{10 \text{ mg}}{10 \text{ mL}} = \frac{3 \text{ mg}}{X \text{ mL}} \qquad \frac{10 \text{ mg}}{10 \text{ mL}} = \frac{3 \text{ mg}}{X \text{ mL}}$$

   $5X = 3 \times 5$                                    $10X = 3 \times 10$
   
   or
   
   $5X = 15$                                    $10X = 30$

5. **Divide**

   $5X = 15$                                    $10X = 30$

   $$X = \frac{15}{5} \qquad\qquad\text{or}\qquad\qquad X = \frac{30}{10}$$

   $X = 3 \text{ mL}$                                    $X = 3 \text{ mL}$

**In summary, give Claritin Syrup 3 mg to the child, 3 mL should be given.**

**Note:** *Measure this with a 3 mL syringe for accuracy.*

# Oral Medications

Directions: The orders are written as the physician would write it on the order sheet. Calculate the following problems for the first dose of the day.

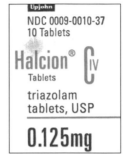

1. The doctor orders Halcion (triazolam) 0.25 mg po HS prn sleep.
   Read the label. What would you give?　————

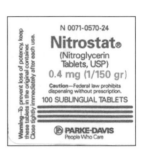

2. The doctor orders Nitrostat (nitroglycerin). 0.4 mg sublingual (under the tongue).
   Read the label. What would you give?　————

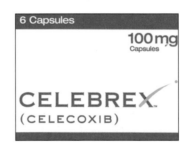

3. The doctor orders Celebrex (celecoxib) 200 mg po qd.
   Read the label. What would you give?　————

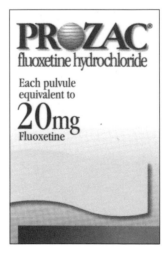

4. The doctor orders Prozac (fluoxetine) 40 mg po qd.
   Read the label. What would you give?　————

5. The doctor orders furosemide 60 mg po bid.
   Read the label. What would you give? _____

**FUROSEMIDE TABLETS, USP**

**40 mg**

100 Tablets (10 x 10)

USUAL DOSAGE: 20 to 80 mg.
See accompanying circular.

6. The doctor orders Dilantin (phenytoin) 200 mg suspension per NG tube qd.
   Read the label. What would you give? _____

**Dilantin-125®**

(Phenytoin Oral Suspension, USP)

**125 mg per 5 mL potency**

**Important**—Another strength available; verify unspecified prescriptions.

**Caution**—Federal law prohibits dispensing without prescription.

7. The doctor orders Micronase (glyburide) 5 mg po qd with breakfast.
   Read the label. What would you give? _____

Upjohn

NDC 0009-0141-11
500 Tablets

**Micronase®**
Tablets

glyburide tablets

**2.5mg**

8. The doctor orders Benadryl (diphenhydramine) 50 mg po q6h prn for itching.
   Read the label. What would you give? _____

**Benadryl®**
(Diphenhydramine HCl Capsules, USP)

**25 mg**

Caution—Federal law prohibits dispensing without prescription.

100 CAPSULES

Ⓟ **PARKE-DAVIS**
People Who Care

9. The doctor orders Lanoxin (digoxin) 0.125 mg p qd.
   Read the label. What would you give? _____

100 Tablets    NDC 0081-0249-55

**LANOXIN®**
(DIGOXIN)
Each scored tablet contains
**250 µg (0.25 mg)**
CAUTION: Federal law prohibits dispensing without prescription.

BURROUGHS WELLCOME CO.
Research Triangle Park, NC 27709

542158

LOT
EXP

For indications, dosage, precautions, etc., see accompanying package insert.
Store at 15° to 25°C (59° to 77°F) in a dry place.
Dispense in tight container as defined in the U.S.P.
6505-00-116-7750    Made in U.S.A.    542158

10. The doctor orders Procardia XL (nifedipine) 60 mg po qd.
    Read the label. What would you give? _____

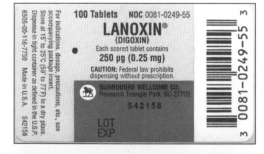

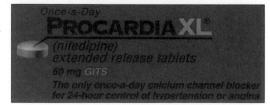

11. The doctor wishes to decrease the dosage of Lanoxin (digoxin). You have two different doses of digoxin.
    Which tablet is a lower dosage?        _____

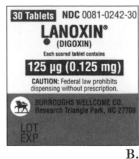

A.                                      B.

12. The doctor orders Potassium Chloride 30 mEq po tid.
    Read the label. What would you give?        _____

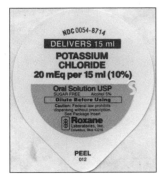

13. The doctor orders Cardizem (diltiazem HCl) 30 mg po qid ac meals and at bedtime.
    Read the label. What would you give?        _____

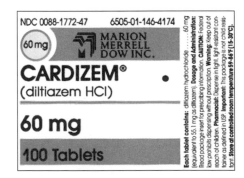

14. The doctor orders Quinaglute Dura-Tab (quinidine gluconate) 324 mg po bid.
    Read the label.
    What would you give?           a. _____
      Is this long or short acting?   b. _____
      Can this tablet be crushed?     c. _____

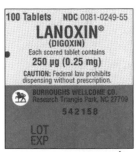

15. The doctor orders Coumadin (sodium warfarin) 5 mg po today.
    Read the label. What would you give?        _____

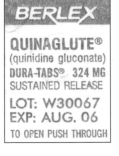

16. The doctor orders Vasotec (enalapril maleate) 20 mg po qd.
    Read the label. What would you give? _____

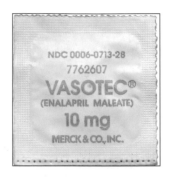

17. The doctor orders Inderal (propranolol) 40 mg po qid.
    Read the label. What would you give? _____

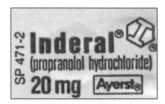

18. The doctor orders Capoten (captopril) 6.25 mg po q8h.
    Read the label. What would you give? _____

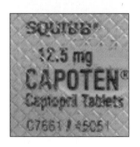

19. The doctor orders Keflex (cephalexin monohydrate) suspen-
    sion 500 mg q6h per gastrostomy tube.
    Read the label. What would you give? _____

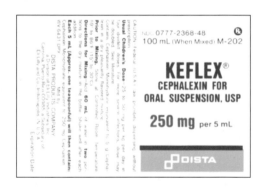

20. The doctor orders quinidine sulfate 150 mg po q8h.
    Read the label. What would you give? _____

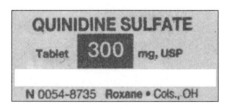

The problems on the next page will give you background information in real life situations. To be successful at solving the problems, look for the relevant information which is what the doctor has ordered, read the drug label, and determine what dosage should be given.

21. Ms. Gray has rheumatoid arthritis. The doctor orders Meclomen (meclofenamate) 150 mg po q6h prn, a non-steroidal anti-inflammatory for her pain.
Read the label. What would you give? _____

N 0071-0268-24
**Meclomen**®
(Meclofenamate Sodium Capsules, USP)
**50 mg**
Caution—Federal law prohibits dispensing without prescription.
**100 CAPSULES**
℗ **PARKE-DAVIS**
People Who Care

22. Ms. James has cystitis accompanied with burning and painful urination. The doctor orders Pyridium (phenazopyridine) 200 mg po tid with meals.
Read the label. What would you give? _____

**Pyridium**®
(Phenazopyridine HCl Tablets, USP)
**100 mg**
Caution—Federal law prohibits dispensing without prescription.
**100 TABLETS**
℗ **PARKE-DAVIS**
People Who Care

23. The doctor orders Easprin (enteric coated aspirin delayed release) 30 grains po bid for Ms. Peterson's arthritic pain.
Read the label. What would you give? _____

**Easprin**®
(Aspirin Delayed-release Tablets, USP)
**Enteric Coated**
**15 grain** (975 mg)
Caution—Federal law prohibits dispensing without prescription.
**100 TABLETS**
℗ **PARKE-DAVIS**
People Who Care

24. The doctor orders Levothroid (levothyroxine sodium) 150 mcg po qd for thyroid replacement therapy.
Read the label. What would you give? _____

UNIT DOSE    NDC 0456-0323-63
**Levothroid**®
**Tablets**
(levothyroxine sodium tablets, USP)
**100 mcg**
100 TABLETS – 10 strips of 10

25. The doctor orders Imuran (azathioprine) 75 mg po bid following Mr. Blain's kidney transplant for immuno-suppressant therapy.
Read the label. What would you give? _____

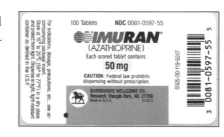

100 Tablets    NDC 0081-0597-55
**IMURAN**®
(AZATHIOPRINE)
Each scored tablet contains
**50 mg**
CAUTION: Federal law prohibits dispensing without prescription.
BURROUGHS WELLCOME CO.
Research Triangle Park, NC 27709
Made in U.S.A.

Answers: Chapter 2, 1-25

| | | | | | |
|---|---|---|---|---|---|
| 1. 2 tablets | 6. 8 mL | 11. B-0.125 | 16. 2 tablets | 21. 3 tablets |
| 2. 1 tablet | 7. 2 tablets | 12. 22.5 mL | 17. 2 tablets | 22. 2 tablets |
| 3. 2 tablets | 8. 2 tablets | 13. 0.5 tablet | 18. 0.5 tablet | 23. 2 tablets |
| 4. 2 tablets | 9. 0.5 tablet | 14. a. 1 tablet b. long acting c. No | 19. 10 mL | 24. 1.5 tablets |
| 5. 1.5 tablets | 10. 1 tablet | 15. 2 tablets | 20. 0.5 tablet | 25. 1.5 tablets |

# Injectable Drugs

Injectable drugs or parenteral drugs are given through intramuscular, intravenous or subcutaneous routes. The drug is placed in a solution for administration and the dosage is measured in milliliters.

Total amount in the vial may differ from the amount per mL. Notice that the quinidine gluconate vial is a multiple dose vial. On the label it states that there are 80 mg per mL, but the vial contains a total 10 mL or 800 mg.

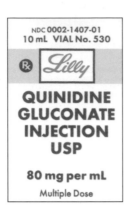

The Solu - Medrol Label is a single dose vial with 40 mg/mL.

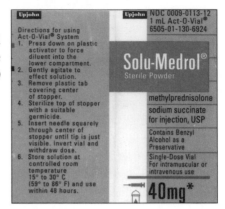

### Route for parenteral drugs

Many drug labels for parenteral use state on the label the route the drug may be given. The SoluMedrol label states it can be used for IM or IV use. Find out if the drug that is available may be given the route that is specified. Example: Regular insulin is the only type of insulin that may be given IV. Procaine Penicillin G may only be given IM. Sus-Phrine may only be given subcutaneously. Read the label and be sure you have the right form of the drug for the prescribed route.

### Diluted versus straight IV push

Some drugs may be drawn up directly from the vial such as furosemide, and given IV push. Other drugs such as antibiotics and potassium chloride must be drawn up from the vial and further diluted with an appropriate solution. Never give a drug straight push that must be further diluted and titrated over time.

### Time over which a drug may be given

Drugs given IV push have a minimum amount of time over which the drug may be given. Determine this rate before giving any drug IV push. Example: Atropine 1 mg must be given over 12 minutes, Valium 5 mg over 1 minute, and Dilantin 50 mg over one minute. Speed shock can occur when a drug is infused too rapidly. High concentrations of the drug reach the heart and brain causing headache, tightness of the chest, drop in blood pressure, or cardiac arrest. Drugs diluted for IV piggyback administration must be given over 15 minutes to 1 hour depending on the drug. Example: Flagyl must be given in 100 mL over 1 hour, and tobramycin must be given in 50-100 mL over 20-60 minutes.

### Compatibility of more than one drug given at the same time

Many drugs are totally incompatible with other drugs and so may not be administered in the same IV tubing. Drugs should never be administered with blood or TPN (total parental nutrition). If the patient will need to receive an IV PB while blood is infusing, it will be necessary to start a separate IV. When patients are receiving multiple IV drugs, the multilumen catheter allows for a separate line for each drug. When giving IV push drugs, such as Valium or Dilantin, use the port most proximal to the insertion site of the IV. These drugs have limited solubility in water. Using the proximal site provides minimal time for the drug to mix with the IV solution. Occasionally it will be necessary to give more than one drug in an IV line. Always check with a current drug handbook or a pharmacist to be certain the drugs are compatible. If they are not compatible, start a second IV.

# Injectable Drugs *cont.*

### Patency of IV

Before giving an IV push or IV PB, check the IV site to be sure there is no redness, no swelling, and no pain. Next check to make sure the medication is compatible with what is in the primary IV bag. Then, give the medication according to hospital policy.

### Patency of Saline Lock

Before giving an IV piggyback or IV push into a saline lock, always check the saline lock for patency. This can be accomplished by aspirating and then injecting 2-3 mL of sodium chloride for injection into the catheter. Indications that the catheter is patent are a blood return with aspiration, and lack of resistance with injection. In addition there should be no pain, no redness and no swelling at the IV site.

### Observe for Adverse Reactions of the drug

When a drug is given as an IV push, the effect is immediate. Be alert to possible adverse effects of the drug and observe the patient closely. Stay with the patient at least 5 minutes after the drug has been given. Should adverse effects occur, stop the drug, check the vital signs, and notify the physician immediately.

# Method:  Ratio Proportion
# Injectable Drugs

1. Determine what you are to give (from the physician's order).
2. Determine what is available from the pharmacy by reading the label.
3. Arrange into a ratio proportion with like units in the numerator and like units in the  denominator.
4. Cross-multiply.
5. Divide.

■ *The doctor ordered  Demerol (meperidine) 35 mg IM q4h prn for pain.*

1. **How much Demerol should be given to the patient?**

 Answer:  Demerol 35 mg

2. **What is available from the pharmacy?**

 Answer:  Demerol 100 mg. per mL

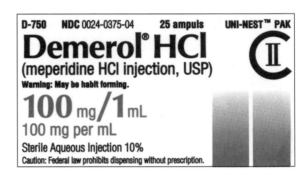

3. **Arrange into a ratio proportion.**

$$\frac{\text{Demerol 100 mg}}{\text{per 1 mL}} = \frac{35 \text{ mg}}{\text{X mL}}$$

To arrange the ratio proportion correctly, like units must be placed on the top and like units placed on the bottom.

Correct

$$\frac{100 \text{ mg}}{1 \text{ mL}} = \frac{35 \text{ mg}}{\text{X mL}} \quad \frac{\text{mg on the top}}{\text{mL on the bottom}}$$

Incorrect

$$\frac{100 \text{ mg}}{1 \text{ mL}} = \frac{\text{X mL}}{35 \text{ mg}}$$

mg and mL mixed on the top

mg and mL mixed on the bottom

**Sample Problem** *cont.*

4      Always place the amount that is available from the pharmacy in a fraction.

Correct

$$\frac{\text{Demerol } 100 \text{ mg}}{\text{per} \quad 1 \text{ mL}}$$

Incorrect

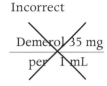

$$\frac{\text{Demerol } 35 \text{ mg}}{\text{per} \quad 1 \text{ mL}}$$

5.      **Cross-multiply**

$$\frac{100 \text{ mg}}{1 \text{ mL}} = \frac{35 \text{ mg}}{\text{X mL}} \qquad \frac{100 \text{ mg}}{1 \text{ mL}} = \frac{35 \text{ mg}}{\text{X mL}}$$

$$100 \text{ X} = 35$$

**Note:** *Always label the units. The answer will be in the units labeled by the X.*

6.      **Divide**

$$\text{X} = \frac{35}{100}$$

$$\text{X} = 0.35 \text{ mL}$$

**Note:** *Always write the unit designation with your answer.*

**Note:** *It is not necessary to round off to 0.4 mL because 0.35 mL can be measured in a TB syringe. See page 114-115 on rules for rounding off.*

■ In summary, mathematically, you are dividing both sides of the equation by the same number. This makes the left side 1 X or X. Practically, divide the left, or X side of the equal sign into the right side of the equal sign.

# Method: Ratio Proportion
# or S Q with more than 1 mL.

*The physician orders digoxin 0.125 mg IM qd. The ampule is labeled 0.5 mg per 2 mL Give_____ mL.*

1.   How much digoxin are you to give this patient?

     Answer: digoxin 0.125 mg

2.   What is available from the pharmacy?

     Answer: digoxin 0.5 mg per 2 mL of solution.

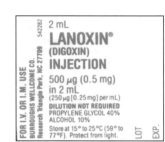

3.   **Arrange ratio proportion**

$$\frac{0.5 \text{ mg}}{2 \text{ mL}} = \frac{0.125 \text{ mg}}{X \text{ mL}}$$

4.   **Cross-multiply**

$$\frac{0.5 \text{ mg}}{2 \text{ mL}} = \frac{0.125 \text{ mg}}{X \text{ mL}} \qquad\qquad \frac{0.5 \text{ mg}}{2 \text{ mL}} = \frac{0.125 \text{ mg}}{X \text{ mL}}$$

0.5 x X = 0.125 x 2

0.5 X = 0.25

5.   **Divide**

$$\frac{0.5X}{0.5} = \frac{0.25}{0.5}$$

X = 0.5 mL

In summary, Digoxin 0.125 mg is contained in 0.5 mL of solution. Draw up 0.5 mL of solution from the ampule.

# Method: Ratio Proportion
# Apothecary with a Fraction

*The doctor orders atropine gr 1/150 IM on call to surgery. Label reads atropine gr 1/200 per 2 mL.*

1. **How much atropine should be given to the patient?**

   Answer: atropine gr 1/150

2. **Find the number of grains per 2 mL from pharmacy.**

   Answer: atropine gr 1/200 per 2 mL of solution.

3. **Arrange ratio proportion**
   $$\frac{1/200 \text{ gr}}{2 \text{ mL}} = \frac{1/150 \text{ gr}}{X \text{mL}}$$

4. **Cross multiply**
   $$\frac{1/200 \text{ gr}}{2 \text{ mL}} = \frac{1/150 \text{gr}}{X \text{ mL}} \qquad \frac{1/200 \text{ gr}}{2 \text{ mL}} = \frac{1/150 \text{ gr}}{X \text{ mL}}$$

   $$1/200 \text{ x } X = 1/150 \text{ x } 2$$

   $$\frac{1}{200} X = \frac{2}{150}$$

5. **Divide**
   $$X = \frac{2}{150} \div \frac{1}{200}$$

   **Invert to divide (To divide a fraction invert and multiply)**

   $$X = \frac{2}{150} \text{ x } \frac{200}{1} = \frac{400}{150}$$

   $$X = \frac{400}{150}$$

   $$X = 2.7 \text{mL}$$

In summary, atropine gr 1/150 is contained in 2.7 mL of solution. Draw up 2.7 mL from the vial.

# Method: Ratio Proportion
# Injectable with Multiple Dose

*The doctor orders Reglan 2.5 mg IV now. Read the label.*

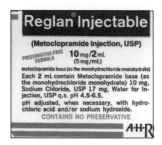

10 mg per 2 mL is the total amount of drug in solution in this vial.
5 mg / mL is the amount of the drug in one mL
When you calculate the dosage, either dosage can be used.

---

**Example: Using multiple dose from label (Reglan 10 mg/2 mL)**

$$\frac{10 \text{ mg}}{2 \text{ mL}} = \frac{2.5 \text{ mg}}{X \text{ mL}}$$

$$10 \, X = 2.5 \times 2$$

$$10 \, X = 5$$

$$X = 0.5 \text{ mL}$$

---

or

---

**Example: Using unit dose from label (Reglan 5 mg / mL)**

$$\frac{5 \text{ mg}}{1 \text{ mL}} = \frac{2.5 \text{ mg}}{X \text{ mL}}$$

$$5 \, X = 2.5$$

$$X = 0.5 \text{ mL}$$

---

In summary, you can use the multiple part of the label or the unit part of the label. From the two examples above, the answer comes out the same which is 0.5 mL. To give 2.5 mg to the patient, 0.5 mL should be given.  0.5 mL = 2.5 mg.

## Injectable Drugs

26. Mr. Jacobsen is scheduled for surgery. The doctor orders promethazine 25 mg IM one hour prior to surgery.
Read the label. Prepare? _____

25 DOSETTE® AMPULS     Each co
NDC 0641-**1496-35**
**PROMETHAZINE**
HCl INJECTION, USP
**50 mg/mL**
**FOR DEEP INTRAMUSCULAR USE ONLY**
Each mL contains promethazine hydrochloride 50 mg, edetate disodium 0.1 mg, calcium chloride 0.04 mg, sodium metabisulfite 0.25 mg and phenol 5 mg in Water for Injection. pH 4.0-5.5; buffered with acetic acid-sodium acetate. Sealed under nitrogen. **USUAL DOSAGE:** See package insert. **PROTECT FROM LIGHT:** Keep covered in carton until time of use. Store at 15°-30°C (59°-86°F).
**DO NOT USE IF SOLUTION HAS DEVELOPED COLOR OR CONTAINS A PRECIPITATE.**
To open ampuls, ignore color line; break at constriction.
Caution: Federal law prohibits dispensing without prescription.
Product Code: 1496-35              8-51496d
**eSi** ELKINS-SINN, INC. Cherry Hill, N

27. Mrs. Weber's BP is 200/105. The doctor orders Vasotec (enalaprilat) 1 mg IV push q6h to be given over 5 minutes duration.
Read the label. Prepare? _____

MSD   NDC 0006-3508-04
**2 mL INJECTION**
**VASOTEC® I.V.**
**(ENALAPRILAT)**
1.25 mg per mL
(Anhydrous equivalent)
**FOR INTRAVENOUS USE ONLY**
CAUTION: Federal (USA) law prohibits dispensing without prescription.
MERCK SHARP & DOHME
DIVISION OF MERCK & CO., INC.
WEST POINT, PA 19486, USA
**1.25 mg per mL**

28. Mr. Houston has a history of atrial fibrillation. The doctor orders quinidine gluconate 200 mg IM q8h.
Read the label. Prepare? _____

NDC 0002-1407-01
10 mL VIAL No. 530
℞ *Lilly*
**QUINIDINE GLUCONATE INJECTION USP**
**80 mg per mL**
Multiple Dose

29. Mr. Juneau has been having frequent PVC's (premature ventricular contractions) that have not responded to lidocaine. The doctor orders Bretylol (bretylium tosylate) 350 mg IV now.
Read the label. Prepare? _____

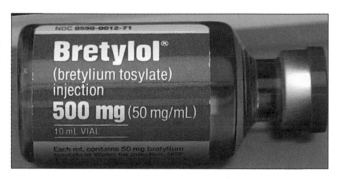

NDC 0590-0012-71
**Bretylol®**
(bretylium tosylate) injection
**500 mg** (50 mg/mL)
10 mL VIAL

30. Mrs. Blaire's heart rate is 200. The doctor orders verapamil 2.5 IV prn heart rate greater than 170. Read the label. Prepare? _____

31. Mrs. Grange has been given a narcotic for pain. Suddenly you notice her respirations have dropped to 6 per minute and she is hard to arouse. You notify the doctor and he orders Narcan (naloxone HCL) 0.2 mg q 3 min x 3 prn to reverse the narcotic.
    Read the label. Prepare?           a. _____
    How many doses may be given?       b. _____

32. Mrs. Bower is having chest pain. The physician orders morphine sulfate 4 mg IV now.
    Read the label. Prepare? _____

33. Mr. Adams becomes very nauseated in the recovery room post operatively. The physician orders Reglan (metoclopramide HCl) 8 mg IV now.
    Read the label. Prepare? _____

34. Mr. Jackson has a gram negative infection. The physician orders gentamicin 50 mg IM q12h.
    Read the label. Prepare? _____

35. Mr. Miller is about to have a heart catheterization. The doctor orders Versed (midazolam HCl) 2.5 mg IV now for sedation.
Read the label. Prepare? _____

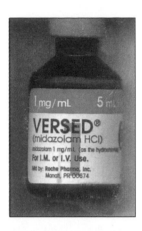

36. After Mr. Miller received the Versed, he has periods of apnea. The doctor orders Romazicon (flumazenil) 0.2 mg IV now to reverse the sedation of the Versed.
Read the label. Prepare? _____

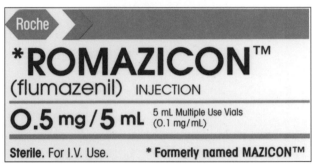

37. Mrs. Meyers had an acute myocardial infarction. The doctor orders Lopressor (metoprolol tartrate) 4 mg IV push over 2 minutes. Repeat x 2 prn.
Read the label. Prepare?        a._____
How many doses may be given?   b._____

38. Mrs. Jones has come to the Emergency Room with hives all over the upper part of her body. The doctor orders Benadryl (diphenhydramine ) 80 mg IM now.
Read the label. Prepare? _____

39. Mr. Blough has been admitted for alcohol abuse. His physician orders thiamine HCl 75 mg IM qd.
    Read the label. Prepare? _____

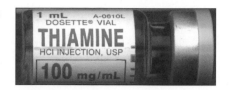

40. The doctor has ordered Phenergan (promethazine HCl) 50 mg IM q6h prn for Mrs. Brown who has been vomiting.
    Read the label. Prepare? _____

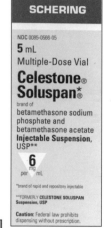

41. Mr. VanOtter has a rash. The physician orders Celestone 7 mg IM now.
    Read the label. Prepare? _____

42. Mr. Smith has aspiration pneumonia. The physician orders Solu Medrol (methylprednisolone sodium succinate) 60 mg IV q6h.
    Read the label. Prepare?          a. _____
    How many vials will you need?     b. _____

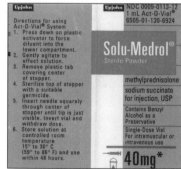

43. Mrs. Clark is in the recovery room. She becomes nauseated and vomits. The doctor orders Inapsine (droperidol) 0.625 mg IV push prn nausea and vomiting, may repeat x 2.
    Read the label. Prepare?
    What type of syringe would you use?   a. _____
    How many doses may be given?          b. _____
                                          c. _____

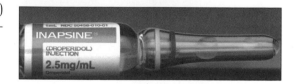

44. Mr. Gonzales has edema of the ankles. The doctor orders furosemide 30 mg IV q12h.
Read the label. Prepare? _____

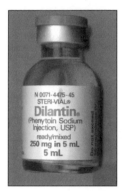

45. Mrs. Schultz has a history of seizures. The doctor orders Dilantin (phenytoin) 200 mg IV bid.
Read the label. Prepare? _____

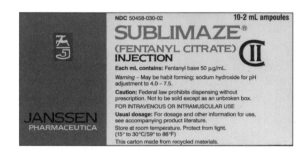

46. Mrs. Hicks is about to have surgery. The doctor orders Sublimaze (fentanyl citrate) 70 mcg IM 30 minutes prior to surgery.
Read the label. Prepare? _____

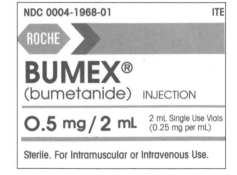

47. Mr. Goldman's output has been low for the last four hours. The doctor orders Bumex (bumetanide) 2 mg IV stat.
Read the label. Prepare? _____

48. Mrs. Castle is complaining of pain following abdominal surgery while in the recovery room. The doctor orders Demerol (meperidine) 8 mg IV q 15 minutes x 3 prn.
Read the label. Prepare?  a. _____
How many doses of Demerol may you give without further orders?  b. _____

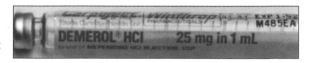

49. Mrs. Hayashi has a history of hypertension. The physician orders hydralazine 30 mg IV q6h prn for a systolic blood pressure greater than 170. Her blood pressure is180 systolic.
Read the label. Prepare? _____

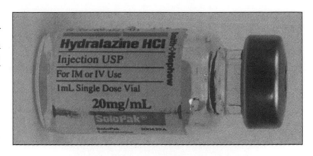

50. Your patient complains of post operative nausea. The doctor orders Compazine (prochlorperazine edisylate) 7.5 mg IM q6h prn nausea.
Read the label. Prepare? _____

51. Mrs. Smith is a frail 95 lb women with pain in her left hip. The doctor orders Morphine 3 mg IV q3h prn for pain.
Read the label. Prepare? _____

52. Mrs. James has a duodenal ulcer. The doctor orders Tagamet (cimetidine) 400 mg IV PB in 100 mL D5W bid. You need to add the Tagamet to a 100 mL bag of D5W.
a. Read the label. Prepare? _____

b. How many vials are needed? _____

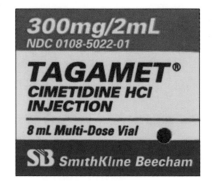

53. Mr. Reyes is to have surgery. The doctor orders Ancef (cefazolin sodium) 750 mg IV PB one hour preoperatively. You will add 750 mg to a 50 mL bag of NS.
Read the label. Prepare?  _____

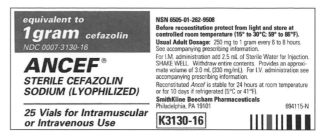

equivalent to
**1gram** cefazolin
NDC 0007-3130-16
**ANCEF®**
**STERILE CEFAZOLIN**
**SODIUM (LYOPHILIZED)**
**25 Vials for Intramuscular**
**or Intravenous Use**  **K3130-16**

NSN 6505-01-262-9508
**Before reconstitution protect from light and store at controlled room temperature (15° to 30°C; 59° to 86°F).**
**Usual Adult Dosage:** 250 mg to 1 gram every 6 to 8 hours.
See accompanying prescribing information.
For I.M. administration add 2.5 mL of Sterile Water for Injection. SHAKE WELL. Withdraw entire contents. Provides an approximate volume of 3.0 mL (330 mg/mL). For I.V. administration see accompanying prescribing information.
Reconstituted *Ancef* is stable for 24 hours at room temperature or for 10 days if refrigerated (5°C or 41°F).
**SmithKline Beecham Pharmaceuticals**
Philadelphia, PA 19101      694115-N

Each vial was reconstituted with 2.5 mL normal saline. The resultant concentration is 330 mg/mL.

54. Mr. Singer is having frequent PVC (premature ventricular contractions). The doctor orders procainamide 100 mg IV push now over 5 minutes. May repeat x 2 q10 min. if PVC's persist.
a. Read the label. Prepare?  _____
b. How many doses may be given?  _____

**Note:** *It would be difficult to give 100 mg over 2 minutes without diluting it. The 2 mL of procainamide could be drawn into a 10 mL syringe along with 8 mL of normal saline. This would change the concentration to 1000 mg per 10 mL with 100 mg/mL.*

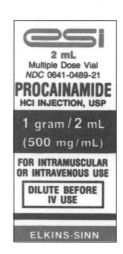

**esi**
2 mL
Multiple Dose Vial
NDC 0641-0489-21
**PROCAINAMIDE**
HCl INJECTION, USP
**1 gram / 2 mL**
**(500 mg/mL)**
**FOR INTRAMUSCULAR**
**OR INTRAVENOUS USE**
**DILUTE BEFORE**
**IV USE**
**ELKINS-SINN**

55. Mrs. Douglas has pneumococci pneumonia. The doctor has ordered 1 million units of penicillin G Procaine IM now.
a. Read the label. Prepare?  _____
b. How much would you discard from the syringe?  _____

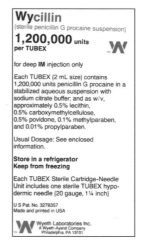

**Wycillin**
(sterile penicillin G procaine suspension)
**1,200,000** units
per TUBEX      **W**

for deep **IM** injection only

Each TUBEX (2 mL size) contains 1,200,000 units penicillin G procaine in a stabilized aqueous suspension with sodium citrate buffer; and as w/v, approximately 0.5% lecithin, 0.5% carboxymethylcellulose, 0.5% povidone, 0.1% methylparaben, and 0.01% propylparaben.

Usual Dosage: See enclosed information.

**Store in a refrigerator**
**Keep from freezing**

Each TUBEX Sterile Cartridge-Needle Unit includes one sterile TUBEX hypodermic needle (20 gauge, 1¼ inch).

U S Pat. No. 3278357
Made and printed in USA

**W** Wyeth Laboratories Inc.
A Wyeth-Ayerst Company
Philadelphia, PA 19101

Answers: Chapter 2,  26-55

| | | | |
|---|---|---|---|
| 26. 0.5 mL | 34. 1.25 or 1.3 mL | 42. a.1.5 mL  b. 2 vials | 49. 1.5 mL |
| 27. 0.8 mL | 35. 2.5 mL | 43. a. 0.25  b. tuberculin | 50. 1.5 mL |
| 28. 2.5 mL | 36. 2 mL | c. 3 | 51. 0.75 mL |
| 29. 7 mL | 37. a.  4 mL   b. 3 | 44. 3 mL | 52. a. 2.66 or 2.7 mL |
| 30. 1 mL | 38. 1.6 mL | 45. 4 mL | b. 1vial |
| 31. a. 0.5 mL b. 3 | 39. 0.75 | 46. 1.4 mL | 53. 2.27 or  2.3 mL |
| 32. 0.4 mL | 40. 2mL | 47. 8 mL | 54. a. 0.2 mL  b. 3 |
| 33. 1.6 mL | 41. 1.2 mL | 48. a. 0.32 mL  b. 3 | 55. a. 1.66 or 1.7 mL  b. 0.3 mL |

# Notes

# 3

# Chapter Three

# Systems
of
Measure

# Systems of Measure

## Introduction
In the health care setting the most commonly used system of measure is the metric system. When doing drug calculation and preparing drugs for administration the metric system should be used. The main focus of this chapter will be the metric system, however, there are two other systems of measures which will be introduced. These systems are the apothecary and the household. Occasionally a drug may be ordered in the apothecary or household measures. Therefore you need to know these systems of measure and how to convert them to the metric system.

## History of Measurements
The history of measurements is an interesting topic. Why measure? Measurements are a part of numerous aspects of our daily life. Just about everything we buy today is measured in one way or another. Measurements tell us such things as the size of a dress or pair of pants, or the volume of milk required for a recipe. Without measurement we could not follow recipes, buy clothes that fit, play organized sports, or build houses.

Primitive people used parts of the body as convenient units of measure, (not standard but always available). Other readily available articles were used including:

INCH   King Edward of England decreed that the inch was the length of three barley corns, round and dry, taken from the center of the ear, and laid end to end.

YARD   The yard can be traced back to the length of the girdle of a Saxon king and comes from the Saxon word "gird," meaning circumference of a person's waist.

FOOT   The term comes from the length of a man's foot.

Measurement is comparison and is only an approximation of the true value of that which is measured. We make many comparisons in our daily lives without even realizing we are doing it; a cat is large compared to a mouse, but small compared to a horse.

## History of Drug Preparation
Drugs were made into powders and brews from plants and herbs. Two examples of those used in pioneer days that grow in the mountains of the West are shown below.

*Purple Gentian*—Grows in high sub-alpine habitat in wet meadows and bogs. Easily identified by its bright purple flowers. The root or chopped herb was steeped, a teaspoon to a cup and drunk 1/2 hour before meals. It was used for chronic indigestion and dyspepsia.

*Prickly Poppy*—Grows in high desert plateaus in the Southwest and in the mountains of New Mexico. The fresh juice from this plant, diluted in three or four parts water was used externally for hives, heat rash, and sunburn.

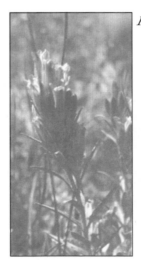

*Purple Gentian*

*Prickly Poppy*

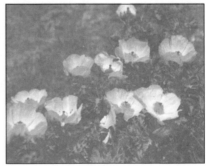

Brewing drugs from plants and herbs was a common practice during the early settlement days of the United States. The information was handed down from generation to generation. The problem in brewing plants and herbs is in standardizing the dosage being taken.

Pharmacology became a science in the 19th century and many of the active constituents of the plants became isolated in a pure form from the plant. Most drugs today are synthetic chemicals with dosages determined by precise weights.

More than one hundred years ago the United States Pharmacopeial Convention adopted the use of the Metric System for measurement of drugs. Today only the metric system of measure should be used for drug calculation. However, it is still possible to find prescriptions written in the apothecary and household systems of measure. All three systems of measurement and their equivalents will be discussed in this chapter so you will know what the prescription means, and if it is in the apothecary or household system you will know how to convert it to the metric system.

## Metric versus Apothecary

Use the metric system for drug calculation and measurement. If a prescription is written in the apothecary or household system, convert the dosage to the metric system.

Be aware that some measuring devices show both systems of measuring. Notice the 3 mL syringe and the tuberculin syringe have both the metric scale in milliliters and the apothecary scale in minims. Use the milliliter scale only and figure the correct dosage in milliliters (mL).

**Use** the scale on the syringe for milliliters

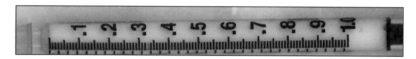

**Do not** use the scale for minims

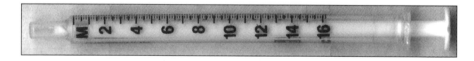

## The Metric System

The metric system is a system of weights and measures which employs kilograms (kg), grams (g), milligrams (mg), micrograms (mcg), liters (L), milliliters (mL), centimeters (cm), and millimeters (mm). The metric system is a decimal based system. Its methods of counting are based on the unit of 10. The decimal system's name is derived from the Latin word decem, meaning ten. It employs zero and nine digits, from which very large and very small numbers can be obtained. Historians of mathematics say the decimal system originated in India, then was revived in Europe via the Arabs and explained exhaustively in 1202 by Leonardo de Pisa, an Italian geometrician. In 1960 the International System of Units (SI) was established for the metric system.

# Metric System of Measure

| Weight | |
|---|---|
| **Unit** | **Equivalents** |
| kilogram (kg) | 1 kg = 1000 g |
| gram (g) | 1 g = 1000 mg |
| milligram (mg) | 1 mg = 1000 mcg<br>1 mg = 0.001 g |
| microgram (mcg) | 1 mcg = 0.001 mg<br>1 mcg = 0.000001 g |

| Volume | |
|---|---|
| **Unit** | **Equivalents** |
| 1 liter (L) | 1 (L) = 1000 mL |
| milliliter (mL) | 1 mL = 1cc<br>1 mL = 0.001 liter |
| cubic centimeter (cc) | 1 cc = 1 mL<br>1 cc = 0.001 liter |

| Length | |
|---|---|
| **Unit** | **Equivalents** |
| meter (M) | 1 M = 1000 mm<br>1 M = 100 cm |
| centimeter (cm) | 1 cm = 10 mm<br>1 cm = 0.01 m |
| millimeter (mm) | 1 mm = 0.1 cm<br>1 mm = 0.001 m |

### Use of the Metric System for Drug Dosage

The metric system uses weight and volume measures for drug calculation. Metric length measures are used to measure height and size of a wound.

> **Gram** is the basic unit of weight
> **milli** means 1/1000  A milligram is one thousandth of a gram
> **micro** means 1/1000,000   A microgram is one millionth of a gram
> **kilo** means 1000  A kilogram is 1000 grams
>
> **Liter** is the basic unit of volume
> **milli** means 1/1000  A milliliter is one thousandth of a liter

### Conversion of units within the metric system

Conversions within the metric system will be frequently encountered. For example the doctor may order Chloral hydrate 0.5 g but the label may read 500 mg per tablet. To calculate the drug dosage, the drug that is ordered and the drug that is available must be in like units. To convert grams to milligrams you multiply by 1000 or move the decimal point three places to the right. 0.5 g = 500 mg. Therefore, you would give 1 tablet.
1 g = 1000 mg or 0.5 g = 500 mg

**Metric Notations:** *Arabic numbers are used*
> *Decimals are used not fractions*
> *The abbreviation for the unit follows the amount - 500 mg*

## Apothecary System of Measures

The apothecary system of measures is an old system brought to the United States from England during the colonial period. It employs grains (gr), pounds (lbs), drams (dr), ounces (oz), pints (pt), and quarts (qt). The origin of the measurement known as grains comes from using grain seeds such as wheat, rice or barley as natural units of weight. The grain is used to represent the smallest unit of troy and avoirdupois weight. The apothecary system is not used very much, however, some physicians do order a few medications such as aspirin in grains. The equivalent of 5 grains is 324 milligrams. Atropine, codeine, and morphine are examples of other drugs that are sometimes ordered in grains.

### Apothecary Notations:

*The number follows the abbreviation.*
*Roman numerals are used. In practice, arabic numbers are also used before the abbreviation.*
*The symbol ss is used for ½ or 0.5*
*Quantities are expressed in fractions not decimals (gr ½)*
*The symbol for fluid dram is* ℨ
*The symbol for fluid ounce is* ℥

Example: **ASPIRIN gr X q4h prn fever > than 101.**
**Note:** *grains comes before the Roman Numeral X*

Example: **Seconal gr iss HS prn sleep**
**Note:** *grains comes before the Roman Numerals iss; iss = 1.5 grains*

| Roman numerals | | Arabic | Roman numerals | | Arabic |
|---|---|---|---|---|---|
| I | i | 1 | VIII | viii | 8 |
| II | ii | 2 | IX | ix | 9 |
| III | iii | 3 | X | x | 10 |
| IV | iv | 4 | XV | xv | 15 |
| V | v | 5 | XX | xx | 20 |
| VI | vi | 6 | XXV | xxv | 25 |
| VII | vii | 7 | C | c | 100 |
| | | | ss | | ½ |

Roman numerals are used with the Apothecary System of Measure.
Aspirin 5 grains is properly written aspirin gr V, using the Roman Numeral for 5.

---

### Apothecary Measures

**Fluid Measures**
60 minims (m) = 1 fluid dram (dr)
8 fluid dram = 1 fluid ounce (oz)
16 fluid ounces = 1 pint (pt)
2 pints (32 fluid ounces) = 1 quart
4 quarts (qt) 8 pints = 1 gallon (gal)

**Weight Measures**
60 grains (gr) = 1 dram (dr)
8 drams (dr) = 1 ounce (oz)

## Apothecary  Metric

### Equivalents

**Fluid Measures**

| | | |
|---|---|---|
| 15 minims | = | 1 milliliter (mL) |
| 1 dram (dr) | = | 4 milliliters (mL) |
| 4 dram | = | 15 milliliters (mL) |
| 8 dram (1 oz) | = | 30 milliliters (mL) |

**Weight Measures**

| | | |
|---|---|---|
| 1 grain (gr) | = | 60 milligrams (mg) |
| 15 grains | = | 1 gram (g) |
| 4 drams | = | 15 grams (g) |

## Relationship of Weight Equivalents

1 kilogram = 1000 grams

1 gram = 1000 milligrams

1 gram = 15 grains

1 grain = 60 milligrams

1 milligram = 1000 micrograms

A kilogram is 1000 times heavier than a gram;
a gram is 15 times heavier than a grain;
a grain is 60 times heavier than a milligram;
a milligram is 1000 times heavier than a microgram.

**Familiar Conversion**

An example of a familiar conversion is 12 inches = 1 foot

If the above stem is known, it is easy to calculate that 24 inches = X feet.

$$\frac{12 \text{ inches}}{1 \text{ foot}} = \frac{24 \text{ inches}}{X \text{ feet}}$$

12x X = 24

$$X = \frac{24}{12}$$

X = 2 feet

## Household Measures

Household measures include measures that are readily available in most homes such as drops, teaspoons, tablespoons, ounce cups, pints, quarts, feet (rulers), and pounds (scales)

| Household | | Metric |
|---|---|---|
| 15 drops | = | 1 milliliter (mL) |
| 1 teaspoon (tsp) | = | 5 milliliters (mL) |
| 3 tsp (1 Tbs) | = | 15 milliliters (mL) |
| 1 tablespoon (Tbs) | = | 15 milliliters (mL) |
| 2 Tbs = (1 oz) | = | 30 milliliters (mL) |
| 1 cup (c) | = | 240 milliliters (mL) |
| 1 pint (pt) | = | 500 milliliters (mL) |
| 1 quart (32) oz | = | 1000 milliliters (mL) |
| **Weight** | | |
| 2.2 pounds (lb) | = | 1 kilogram (kg) |
| **Length** | | |
| 1 inch | = | 2.5 centimeters |
| 1 inch | = | 25 millimeters |

## Ounce Cup

Memorization of the liquid measurements and conversions may be done more easily by examining the ounce cup. Examine the cup and become familiar with the approximate equivalents.

1 oz = 30 mL or 8 dr or 2 Tbs

1 tsp = 5 mL or 1 dr

1/2 oz = 15 mL or 4 dr or 1 Tbs

8 oz = 240 mL or 1 cup

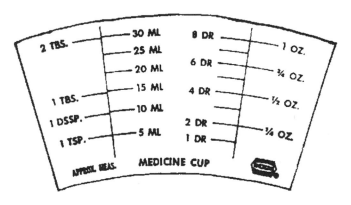

# Conversion Table to be Memorized

Listed on this page is the Conversion Table that must be memorized. One method for memorization is to use flash cards. Put 60 mg = on one side of the card, 1 gr = on the other side of the card. As you do additional problems, the conversions will become more familiar.

The list by no means contains all the stems for conversion from the apothecary or household to the metric system of measures. However, those listed are utilized for the calculation of drug dosages. When you become familiar with, or memorize the table, it is much easier to conceptualize drug problems.

## CONVERSION TABLE

### Metric Volume

1 L = 1000 mL

1 L = 1000 cc

### Metric Weight

1000 mcg = 1 mg

1000 mg = 1 g

1000 g = 1 kg

### Weights: Apothecary/ Household to Metric

1 gr = 60 mg

15 gr = 1 g

2.2 lbs = 1 kg

### Solutions

1 g per 100 cc = 1% solution

25 g per 100 cc = 25% solution

100 g per 100 cc = 100% solution

### Liquids

| | | |
|---|---|---|
| 1 mL = 1 cc | 15 mL = 3 tsp | 2 c = 1 pt |
| 1 mL = 15 gtts | 15 mL = 1 Tbs | 1000 mL = 1 qt |
| 1 mL = 15 minims | 30 mL = 1 oz | 32 oz = 1 qt |
| 1 mL = 60 microdrops | 1 Tbs = 3 tsp | 1 L = 1 qt |
| 4 mL = 1 dr | 8 dr = 1 oz | 1 L = 1000 mL |
| 5 mL = 1 tsp | 240 mL = 1 c | 4 qt = 1 gal |
| | 500 mL = 1 pt | |

**Note:** *The conversion tables give approximate equivalents. These equivalents are not exact. For example, 1 liter = 1 quart. Actually, 1 liter is 1.06 quarts, but for pharmacological purposes they are considered equal. The volume in a drop always depends upon the size of the dropper. Always look at the package (IV tubing, dropper, etc.) to know the correct drop factor. If you are not familiar with the abbreviations, refer to the inside of the front cover.*

# 4

## Chapter Four

# Conversion from One System of Measure to Another

# Conversion from One System
# of Measurement to Another

### Introduction
Chapter 4 presents information on how to convert from apothecary to metric and how to convert within the metric system using the decimal method.

### Conversion from grains to milligrams
When converting from the apothecary system to the metric system, the conversion is never exact. It is an approximate equivalent. For example 60 or 65 milligrams equals 1 grain. Either is acceptable but 60 mg is used more frequently. This is why you see the following variation in drug labels.

| ASPIRIN | ASPIRIN |
| :---: | :---: |
| 300 mg tablet | 325 mg tablet |

Conversion is like translating from one language to another. The translation is not always exactly the same.

When solving mathematical problems you need to know how to convert the units of measure to like terms. In order to do this, examine the following physician's orders. The doctor orders 1/150 grains of atropine. The label is written in milligrams.

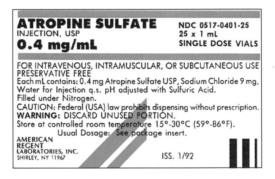

In order to know what to give this patient, you need to convert grains to milligrams. The basic unit of equivalency is 1 grain = approximately 60 milligrams.

### 1 grain = 60 milligrams

The problem must be set up with either grains or milligrams. Because grains has a fraction of 1/150 it makes it easier to convert from grains to milligrams.

Look at the sample problem on page 81. How many milliliters should you prepare?

# Conversion from Apothecary to Metric

■ *The doctor orders atropine gr 1/150 prn for pulse less than 50.*

*The vial is labeled atropine  0.4 mg per 1 mL.*

$$\frac{\text{gr } 1}{60 \text{ mg}} = \frac{\text{gr } 1/150}{X \text{ mg}}$$

See chart for Conversion Table on back cover

$$60 \text{ mg} = 1\text{gr}$$

**ATROPINE SULFATE**
INJECTION, USP
NDC 0517-0401-25
25 x 1 mL
SINGLE DOSE VIALS
**0.4 mg/mL**

FOR INTRAVENOUS, INTRAMUSCULAR, OR SUBCUTANEOUS USE
PRESERVATIVE FREE
Each mL contains: 0.4 mg Atropine Sulfate USP, Sodium Chloride 9 mg,
Water for Injection q.s. pH adjusted with Sulfuric Acid.
Filled under Nitrogen.
CAUTION: Federal (USA) law prohibits dispensing without prescription.
**WARNING:** DISCARD UNUSED PORTION.
Store at controlled room temperature 15°-30°C (59°-86°F).
Usual Dosage:  See package insert.
AMERICAN
REGENT
LABORATORIES, INC.
SHIRLEY, NY 11967
ISS. 1/92

**Cross-multiply**

$$\frac{\text{gr } 1}{60 \text{ mg}} = \frac{\text{gr } 1/150}{X \text{ mg}} \qquad \frac{\text{gr } 1}{60 \text{ mg}} = \frac{\text{gr } 1/150}{X \text{ mg}}$$

$$X = \frac{1}{150} \text{ x } 60$$

$$X = \frac{1}{150} \text{ x } \frac{60}{1}$$

**Divide**

$$\frac{60}{150}$$

$$X = 0.4 \text{ mg}$$

**Note:** *The fraction is eliminated and the answer is in the metric system.*

This type of conversion is used frequently in the work environment. Many of the formulas use kilograms for drug calculation. To work many problems you need to know 1 kg = 2.2 lbs.

■ **In summary, gr 1/150 has been converted to mg.   gr 1/150 = 0.4 mg. Give atropine 1mL**

# Conversion: Apothecary to Metric

▪ *Mrs. Sial weighs 110 pounds.*
    *How many kilograms does she weigh?* _____ *kg.*

### Stem

$$\frac{2.2 \text{ lbs}}{1 \text{ kg}} = \frac{110 \text{ lbs}}{X \text{ kg}}$$

**Note:**  *Like units on top  - lbs*
          *Like units on bottom - kg*

### Cross-multiply

$$\frac{2.2 \text{ lbs}}{1 \text{ kg}} = \frac{110 \text{ lbs}}{X \text{ kg}}$$

$$2.2 \times X = 110$$

$$2.2 \, X = 110$$

### Divide

$$\frac{2.2 \; X}{2.2} = \frac{110}{2.2}$$

$$X = 50 \text{ kg}$$

**Note:** *To change pounds to kilograms, divide pounds by 2.2 (110 ÷ 2.2 = 50 kg).  Until you become very familiar with the conversion of weights, the ratio proportion method is an excellent way to check the answer.*

▪ **In summary, Mrs. Sial weighs 110 lbs or 50 kg**

# Conversion of Percent of Medication to Grams

Percent means parts per hundred. Five percent (5%) is five parts per hundred.
With drugs and solutions, percent is the **number of grams** of the drug **per 100 mL** of solvent.

100 mL of 5% dextrose and water contains 5 g of dextrose
100 mL of 20% Mannitol and water contains 20 g of Mannitol
100 mL of 7.5% of sodium bicarbonate and water contains 7.5 g of sodium bicarbonate.

**How many g of dextrose are there in 1000 mL of D5W?**

$$\frac{5 \text{ g}}{100 \text{ mL}} = \frac{X \text{ g}}{1000 \text{ mL}}$$

$$100 \text{ X} = 5000$$

$$X = 50 \text{ g}$$

■ In summary, 1 liter (1000 mL) of D5W has 50 g of dextrose.

---

# Converting Celsius to Fahrenheit

The patient's temperature is 38.5 C. What is the patient's temperature in Fahrenheit?

**Formula** C° to F° (C x 1.8 ) + 32

38.5°C x 1.8 = 69.3 + 32 = 101.3° F

# Converting Fahrenheit to Celsius

The patient's temperature is 97°. What is the patient's temperature in Celsius?

**Formula F° to C°**

$$\frac{(F - 32)}{1.8}$$

97° - 32 = 65

$$\frac{65}{1.8} = 36° \text{ C}$$

# The Decimal Method of Conversion within the Metric System

**The Metric system is a system of weight and measure based on powers of 10. Since it is a decimal system, conversion between the units is only a matter of moving the decimal point.**

There is a decimal method of doing a conversion within the metric system. The decimal method can only be used in the metric system to convert kg to g, g to mg or mg to mcg. This quick method is possible because each unit is 1000 times the weight of the lighter unit.

How many mg = 0.6 g?

To convert g to mg move the decimal point three places to the right.

g to mg

1 g  = 1000 mg

0.6 g = .600 = 600 mg

To convert **mg** to **g** move the decimal point three places to the left.

mg to g

600 mg = .600. = 0.6 g

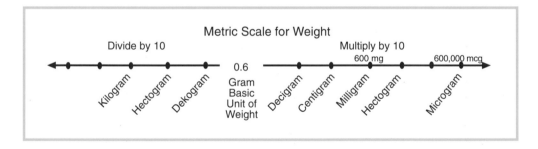

**Note:** *When you move from a g to mg the number will be larger*. Move three spaces to the right. *When you move from mg to g the number will be smaller*. Move three spaces to the left.

If you forget how many places, or which direction, to move the decimal point, use the ratio proportion method of conversion.

$$\frac{1 \text{ g}}{1000 \text{ mg}} = \frac{0.6 \text{ g}}{X \text{ mg}}$$

X = 0.6 x 1000

X = 600 mg

# Conversions

1. gr 1/4 = _____mg

2. gr 7.5 = _____mg

3. 2 tsp = _____mL

4. 60 minims = _____cc

5. gr 1/200 = _____mg

6. 8 oz = _____mL

7. 3 qt = _____mL

8. 100 mg = _____g

9. 100 g  = _____mg

10. 0.25 g = _____mg

11. 45 lbs = _____kg

12. 0.5 mg = _____mcg

13. 45 gtts = _____mL
(package states 15 gtts = 1 cc)

14. gr 20 = _____g

15. 5000 cc = _____L

16. 2500 g = _____kg

17. 2 Tbs = _____mL

18. gr 1/100 = _____mg

19. gr 1/150 = _____mg

20. gr 1/300 = _____mg

21. 150 lbs = _____kg

22. gr  45 = _____g

23. 15 mL = _____cc

24. 5 qt = _____L

25. 4 oz  = _____mL

26. 5 tsp = _____mL

27. dr 8 = _____mL

28. 120 microdrops = _____mL
(package states 60 gtts = 1 cc)

29. 90 microdrops = _____mL
(package states 60 gtts = 1 cc)

30. 60 gtts = _____mL
(package states 15 gtts = 1 cc)

31. 10% solution = _____ g  per 100 cc

32. 15% solution = _____ g  per 10 cc

33. gr 10 = _____mg

34. 2500 mcg = _____mg

35. 15 kg = _____g

36. 2 cc = _____ microdrops
    (package states 60 gtts = 1 cc)

37. 20 kg = _____lbs

38. gr 1/6 = _____mg

39. 25 cc = _____tsp

40. 500 mcg = _____mg

41. 210 lbS = _____kg

42. 125 mcg = _____mg

43. 2 oz = _____mL

44. 20 cc = _____tsp

45. 60 cc = _____T

46. 400 mcg = _____mg

47. 39.5° C = _____° F

48. 98° F = _____° C

Answers: Chapter 4, 1-48

| | | | |
|---|---|---|---|
| 1. 15 mg | 13. 3 mL | 25. 120 mL | 37. 44 lbs |
| 2. 450 mg | 14. 1.3 g(1.33) | 26. 25 mL | 38. 10 mg |
| 3. 10 mL | 15. 5 L | 27. 32 or 30 mL | 39. 5 tsp |
| 4. 4 cc | 16. 2.5 kg | 28. 2 mL | 40. 0.5 mg |
| 5. 0.3 mg | 17. 30 mL | 29. 1.5 mL | 41. 95.45 or 95 kg |
| 6. 240 mL | 18. 0.6 mg | 30. 4 mL | 42. 0.125 mg |
| 7. 3000 mL | 19. 0.4 mg | 31. 10 g per 100 cc | 43. 60 mL |
| 8. 0.1 g | 20. 0.2 mg | 32. 1.5 g per 10 cc | 44. 4 tsp |
| 9. 100,000 mg | 21. 68.2 kg | 33. 600 mg | 45. 4 T |
| 10. 250 mg | 22. 3 g | 34. 2.5 mg | 46. 0.4 mg |
| 11. 20.5 kg(20.454) | 23. 15 cc | 35. 15,000 g | 47. 103.1 F |
| 12. 500 mcg | 24. 5 L | 36. 120 microdrops | 48. 36.6 C |

**5**

Chapter Five

# Drug Calculation Problems Requiring Conversions

# Drug Calculations Requiring Conversions

## Introduction

When a drug is ordered in one measuring system and the dose that is available is supplied in another system, it becomes necessary to convert one of them to make like units.

In the first section of this chapter you will review sample problems of drugs that require conversions and then you will do practice problems that require conversions. In the second part of the chapter you will be given more practice problems. Some will require conversions and some will not. You will need to decide whether the problems need conversions before calculating the dosage. If a conversion is needed, it just requires an extra step. After converting, the problem is done the same as in chapter two for the amount to give.

---

### Things to Consider when Drug Calculation Problems Require Conversions:

1. Look at what is available and what you want to give. Ask yourself the question, "Are the drugs in the same units of measure?"

2. If the drugs are not in the same units of measure, convert one.

3. **It is best to convert to the metric system,** since it is a decimal system and you will not have to deal with fractions.

4. Sometimes you must convert within the same system of measure to make like units. Example: grams to milligrams.

5. Two steps.
   Step A: Convert the dose from the system in which it is ordered to the system in which it is available.
   Step B: Calculate the amount needed to obtain the desired dose.

---

# Problems Requiring a Conversion

■ *The physician has ordered 0.35 g of ampicillin IM.*

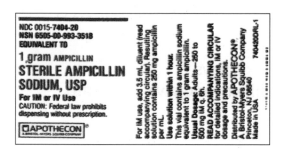

Reconstituted with 3.5 mL of diluent

Step A: Convert the dose from the system in which it is ordered to the system in which it is available.

### 1. How much ampicillin should be given to the patient?

Answer: 0.35 g of ampicillin

### 2. What is available from the pharmacy? Read the label.

Answer: 250 mg of ampicillin per 1 mL

### 3. Are they in the same units?

0.35 g - 250 mg

*Different Units*

Answer: No

### 4. Convert one of them so they are in the same units.

$$\frac{1\,g}{1000\,mg} = \frac{0.35\,g}{X\,mg}$$

$1\,X = 0.35 \times 1000$

$X = 350\,mg$

Answer: 0.35 g = 350 mg or decimal method: 0.35 g = 0.350. mg = 350mg
(move decimal)

Step B: Calculate the amount needed to obtain the desired dose.

### 5. Dosage Calculation: Arrange ratio proportion. Now that you have like units, continue with the problem as if it were the usual calculation problem.

$$\frac{250\,mg}{1\,mL} = \frac{350\,mg}{X\,mL} \qquad 250\,X = 350 \qquad X = 1.4\,mL$$

■ In summary 0.35 g = 350 mg = 1.4 mL  Give 1.4 mL.

# Problems Requiring a Conversion

▪ *A physician ordered morphine sulfate gr 1/8 IM q4h prn for pain.*

Step A: Convert the dose from the system in which it is ordered to the system in which it is available.

   **1. How much morphine sulfate should be given to the patient?**

   Answer: morphine sulfate gr 1/8

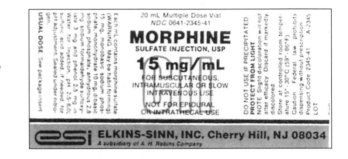

   **2. What is available from the pharmacy?**
   Read the label.

   Answer: morphine sulfate 15 mg/mL

**3. Are the above in like units?**

   Answer: No

   gr 1/8          15 mg / mL

   *Different units*

   **4. Convert one of the above. It is easier to convert to the metric system.**
   This eliminates the fraction.

$$\frac{gr\ 1}{60\ mg} = \frac{gr\ \dfrac{1}{8}}{X\ mg} \qquad\qquad \frac{gr\ 1}{60\ mg} = \frac{gr\ \dfrac{1}{8}}{X\ mg}$$

$$1X = \frac{1}{8} \times 60$$

$$X = \frac{1}{8} \times \frac{60}{1}$$

$$X = \frac{60}{8} \qquad\qquad X = 7.5\ mg \qquad \text{Answer: gr 1/8} = 7.5\ mg \qquad \textit{continued on the next page}$$

Step B: Calculate the amount needed to obtain the desired dose.
**Dosage**

### 5. Arrange ratio proportion

$$\frac{15 \text{ mg}}{1 \text{ mL}} = \frac{7.5 \text{ mg}}{X \text{ mL}}$$

$$15 \text{ X} = 7.5$$

$$\text{X} = \frac{7.5}{15}$$

$$\text{X} = 0.5 \text{ mL}$$

▮ **In summary grains 1/8 = 7.5 mg. 7.5 mg = 0.5 mL. Give 0.5 mL**

### Conversions

1. The physician orders aspirin (ASA) gr 10 po q3h prn. Read the drug label and calculate the correct dosage.

    Prepare _____

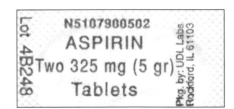

2. The physician orders atropine gr 1/200 IM preoperatively. Read the label and calculate the correct dosage.

    Prepare _____

**ATROPINE SULFATE**
INJECTION, USP
**0.4 mg/mL**
NDC 0517-0401-25
25 x 1 mL
SINGLE DOSE VIALS

FOR INTRAVENOUS, INTRAMUSCULAR, OR SUBCUTANEOUS USE
PRESERVATIVE FREE
Each mL contains: 0.4 mg Atropine Sulfate USP, Sodium Chloride 9 mg,
Water for Injection q.s. pH adjusted with Sulfuric Acid.
Filled under Nitrogen.
CAUTION: Federal (USA) law prohibits dispensing without prescription.
**WARNING:** DISCARD UNUSED PORTION.
Store at controlled room temperature 15°-30°C (59°-86°F).
Usual Dosage: See package insert.
AMERICAN
REGENT
LABORATORIES, INC.
SHIRLEY, NY 11967
ISS. 1/92

3. Mrs. James has been on a daily dose of Levothroid (levothyroxine) 0.1 mg po. Read the label and calculate the correct dosage.

        Prepare _____

UNIT DOSE   NDC 0456-0323-63

**Levothroid®
Tablets**

(levothyroxine sodium tablets, USP)

**100 mcg**

100 TABLETS – 10 strips of 10

4. The physician has ordered chloral hydrate 0.5 g po HS prn for sleep. Read the label and calculate the correct dosage.

        Prepare_____

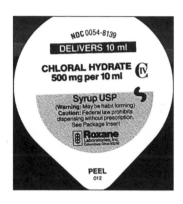

5. The physician orders Lanoxin (digoxin) 0.375 mg IV now. Read the label and calculate the correct dosage.

        Prepare_____

FOR I.V. OR I.M. USE
BURROUGHS WELLCOME CO.
Research Triangle Park, NC 27709  542282

2 mL
**LANOXIN®**
**(DIGOXIN)**
**INJECTION**
500 µg (0.5 mg)
in 2 mL
(250 µg [0.25 mg] per mL)
**DILUTION NOT REQUIRED**
PROPYLENE GLYCOL 40%
ALCOHOL 10%
Store at 15° to 25°C (59° to 77°F). Protect from light.

LOT    EXP.

6. Mrs. Bower is having pain. The physician orders morphine sulfate gr ¼ po q4h prn for pain. Read the label and calculate the correct dosage.

        Prepare _____

NDC 0054-      100 Tablets
4582-25  **15 mg**  Ⓒ

**MORPHINE SULFATE**
**Immediate Release**
**Tablets**

Each tablet contains
Morphine Sulfate 15 mg
(Warning: May be habit forming)
Caution: Federal law prohibits
dispensing without prescription.

Roxane
Laboratories, Inc.
Columbus, Ohio 43216

7. The physician orders codeine sulfate gr 1 po q4h prn for pain. Read the label and calculate the correct dosage.

    Prepare _____

NDC 0054-
4156-25   100 Tablets
**30 mg**   (II)
**CODEINE**
Sulfate
Tablets USP

Each tablet contains Codeine Sulfate 30 mg
(Warning: May be habit forming)
Caution: Federal law prohibits
dispensing without prescription.

Roxane
Laboratories, Inc.
Columbus, Ohio 43216

8. Mrs. Rust is scheduled for surgery. The physician orders fentanyl 0.025 mg IV preoperatively. Read the label and calculate the correct dosage.

    Prepare _____

NDC 50458-030-02   **10-2 mL ampoules**

**SUBLIMAZE®**
**(FENTANYL CITRATE)**   (II)
**INJECTION**

Each mL contains: Fentanyl base 50 μg/mL.

*Warning* – May be habit forming; sodium hydroxide for pH adjustment to 4.0 – 7.5.

**Caution:** Federal law prohibits dispensing without prescription. Not to be sold except as an unbroken box.

FOR INTRAVENOUS OR INTRAMUSCULAR USE

**Usual dosage:** For dosage and other information for use, see accompanying product literature.

Store at room temperature. Protect from light.
(15° to 30°C/59° to 86°F)

This carton made from recycled materials.

9. The physician orders Vitamin C (Ascorbic Acid) 1 g po qd for Mrs. Lorenzen. Read the label and calculate the correct dosage.

    Prepare _____

**VITAMIN C**
**(ASCORBIC ACID)**
**TABLETS**
**500 mg**
**100 Tablets (10 x 10)**
Protect product from light.
Do not expose to excessive heat or moisture.

10. Mrs. Jansen has a seizure disorder. The physician has ordered phenobarbital gr $\frac{1}{2}$ po tid. Read the label and calculate the correct dosage.

    Prepare _____

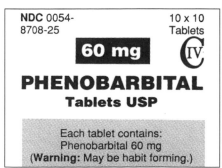

NDC 0054-   10 x 10
8708-25   Tablets
**60 mg**   (IV)
**PHENOBARBITAL**
**Tablets USP**

Each tablet contains:
Phenobarbital 60 mg
(**Warning:** May be habit forming.)

11. The physician has ordered acetaminophen gr X oral solution per NG tube q4h prn for mild pain. Read the label and calculate the correct dosage.

    Prepare _____

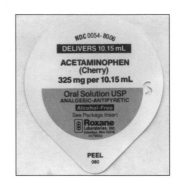

12. The physician orders Keflex (cephalexin monohydrate) 0.5 g per NG tube q6h. Read the label and calculate the correct dosage.

    Prepare _____

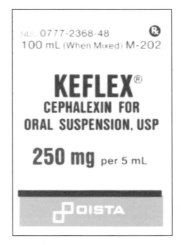

13. The physician orders Lanoxin (digoxin) 0.25 mg po qd. Read the label and calculate the correct dosage.

    Prepare _____

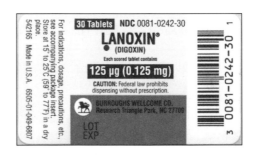

14. The physician orders Tylenol # 3 (acetaminophen gr V and codeine gr ss combined) po q4h prn for pain. Read the label and calculate the correct dosage.

    Prepare_____

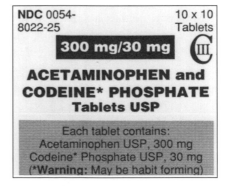

15. The physician orders levothyroxine 0.3 mg IV qd. Read the label and calculate the correct dosage.

     A. Prepare _____

     B. How many vials are needed?
     _____

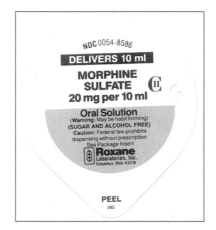

NDC 51079-706-01

**LEVOTHYROXINE SODIUM FOR INJECTION**

**200 mcg**

FOR IM OR IV USE ONLY

Mfg. by BVL., INC. Bedford, OH 44146

Dist. by **UDL** LABS., INC. Rockford, IL 61103

VIAL CONTAINS 200 mcg LEVOTHY-ROXINE SODIUM, 10 mg MANNITOL, 0.7 mg TRIBASIC SODIUM PHOSPHATE, AND SODIUM HYDROXIDE FOR pH ADJUSTMENT.

USUAL DOSE: 200-500 mcg. SEE INSERT FOR COMPLETE INFORMATION.

USE IMMEDIATELY AFTER RECONSTITUTION WITH 5 ML OF 0.9% SODIUM CHLORIDE INJECTION, USP ONLY. PRESERVATIVE FREE. DISCARD ANY UNUSED PORTION.

Reconstituted with 5 mL of preservative free sodium chloride.

16. The physician orders morphine sulfate gr ¼ po q4h prn for pain. Read the label and calculate the correct dosage.

     Prepare _____

NDC 0054-8586

**DELIVERS 10 ml**

**MORPHINE SULFATE** C-II
**20 mg per 10 ml**

**Oral Solution**
(Warning: May be habit forming)
(SUGAR AND ALCOHOL FREE)
Caution: Federal law prohibits dispensing without prescription.
See Package Insert

**Roxane** Laboratories, Inc.
Columbus, Ohio 43216

**PEEL**
065

17. The physician orders Solu-Medrol (methylprednisolone) 0.5 g IV now. Read the label and calculate the correct dosage.

     Prepare _____

Single-Dose Vial    For intramuscular or intravenous use. See package insert for complete product information. Contains Benzyl Alcohol as a Preservative. Store solution at controlled room temperature 15° to 30° C (59° to 86° F) and use within 48 hours after mixing. Each 4 mL (when mixed) contains: methylprednisolone sodium succinate equivalent to 500 mg methylprednisolone (125 mg per mL). Lyophilized in container.                813 974 102
The Upjohn Company • Kalamazoo, MI 49001, USA

NDC 0009-0765-02          4 mL Act-O-Vial®

**Solu-Medrol®** Sterile Powder
methylprednisolone sodium succinate for injection, USP

**500 mg***

18. The physician orders Ilosone (erythromycin) suspension gr viiss per NG tube q6h. Read the label and calculate the correct dosage.

     Prepare _____

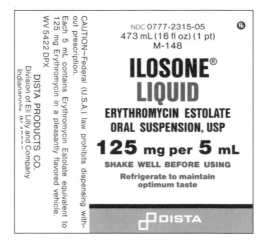

CAUTION—Federal (U.S.A.) law prohibits dispensing without prescription.
Each 5 mL contains Erythromycin Estolate equivalent to 125 mg Erythromycin in a pleasantly flavored vehicle.

DISTA PRODUCTS CO.
Division of Eli Lilly and Company
Indianapolis, IN
WV 5422 DPX

NDC 0777-2315-05
473 mL (16 fl oz) (1 pt)
M-148

**ILOSONE®**
**LIQUID**
**ERYTHROMYCIN ESTOLATE ORAL SUSPENSION, USP**

**125 mg per 5 mL**
SHAKE WELL BEFORE USING
**Refrigerate to maintain optimum taste**

**DISTA**

19. The physician orders codeine gr ¼ po q4h prn for pain. Read the label and calculate the correct dosage.

    Prepare _____

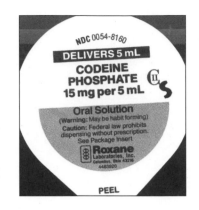

20. The physician orders amoxicillin gr ii po q6h. Read the label and calculate the correct dosage.

    Prepare _____

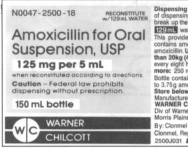

## Problems Requiring / Not Requiring Conversions

Some of the following problems require conversions while others do not. Think about the problems and decide whether a conversion is needed, then work the problem.

21. The physician orders Thorazine (chlorpromazine) 30 mg IM q3h prn agitation. Read the label and calculate the correct dosage.

    Prepare _____

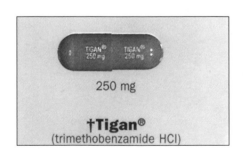

22. The physician orders Tigan (trimethobenzamide) 0.25 g po for nausea. Read the label and calculate the correct dosage.

    Prepare _____

23. The physician orders morphine sulfate gr 1/6 IM q4h prn for pain. Read the label and calculate the correct dosage.

    Prepare _____

    25 DOSETTE® Vials
    Each contains **1 mL**
    **MORPHINE** C II
    SULFATE INJECTION, USP
    **10 mg/mL** WARNING: May be habit forming.
    FOR SC, IM OR SLOW IV USE
    NOT FOR EPIDURAL OR INTRATHECAL USE
    PROTECT FROM LIGHT — Store at 15°-30°C (59°-86°F). Avoid freezing.
    USUAL DOSAGE: See package insert.

    NDC 0641-**0180-25**
    Each mL contains morphine sulfate 10 mg, monobasic sodium phosphate, monohydrate 10 mg, dibasic sodium phosphate, anhydrous 2.8 mg, sodium formaldehyde sulfoxylate 3 mg and phenol 2.5 mg in Water for Injection. pH 2.5-6.5; sulfuric acid added, if needed, for pH adjustment. Sealed under nitrogen. NOTE: Do not use if color is darker than pale yellow, if it is discolored in any other way or if it contains a precipitate. Caution: Federal law prohibits dispensing without prescription. Code: 0180-25 B-50180h

    ELKINS-SINN, INC. Cherry Hill, NJ 08003-4099
    A subsidiary of A. H. Robins Company

24. The physician orders Pitocin (oxytocin) 15 units to be added to 1000 mL D5NS to control post partum bleeding. Read the label and calculate the correct dosage.

    Prepare _____

    N 0071-4160-03
    **Pitocin®**
    (Oxytocin Inj, USP)
    *Synthetic*
    **10 units 1 mL**
    **PARKE-DAVIS**
    **4160G034**

25. The physician orders Chloromycetin (chloramphenicol) 800 mg IV per soluset. Read the label and calculate the correct dosage.

    Prepare _____

    N 0071-4057-03
    **Chloromycetin®**
    **Sodium Succinate**
    (Sterile Chloramphenicol Sodium Succinate, USP)
    Each vial delivers the equivalent of
    **1 GRAM** chloramphenicol
    **100 mg per mL** when reconstituted
    Caution—Federal law prohibits dispensing without prescription.
    **P** **PARKE-DAVIS**
    People Who Care

    Warning—Blood dyscrasias may be associated with the use of chloramphenicol. It is essential that adequate blood studies be made. See enclosed warnings and precautions.
    For intravenous administration.
    Usual Adult Daily Dose—50 mg per kg. See package insert.
    Contents have been freeze-dried in vial.
    Store between 15° and 25°C (59° and 77°F). Keep this and all drugs out of the reach of children.
    To prepare a 10% (100 mg/mL) solution, add 10 mL of sterile aqueous diluent such as Sterile Water for Injection or 5% Dextrose Injection. When reconstituted as directed, 10 mL contains the equivalent of 1 gram chloramphenicol.
    Solution may be kept at room temperature and should be used within 30 days. A cloudy solution should not be used.
    **PARKE-DAVIS**
    Div of Warner-Lambert Co. ©1993
    Morris Plains, NJ 07950 USA

    Reconstituted with 10mL of sterile water.

26. The physician orders Trandate (labetalol) 20 mg IV push over 2 minutes to quickly lower Mr. Swanson's blood pressure. Read the label and calculate the correct dosage.

    Prepare _____

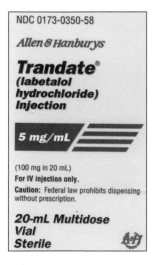

    NDC 0173-0350-58
    *Allen & Hanburys*
    **Trandate®**
    **(labetalol hydrochloride)**
    **Injection**
    **5 mg/mL**
    (100 mg in 20 mL)
    For IV injection only.
    Caution: Federal law prohibits dispensing without prescription.
    **20-mL Multidose Vial Sterile**

27. The physician orders morphine gr ¼ SQ q4h prn for pain. Read the label and calculate the correct dosage.

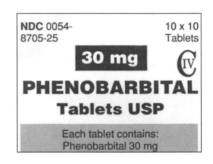

Prepare _____

28. The physician orders phenobarbital gr i po q12h. Read the label and calculate the correct dosage.

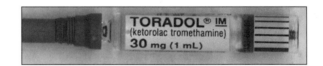

Prepare _____

29. The physician orders Toradol (ketorolac) gr ss IM q6h prn for pain. Read the label and calculate the correct dosage.

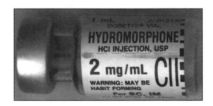

Prepare_____

30. The physician orders Dilaudid (hydromorphone) 0.25 mg IV now. Read the label and calculate the correct dosage.

Prepare _____

Answers: Chapter 5, 1-30

| | | | |
|---|---|---|---|
| 1. 2 tablets | 9. 2 tablets | 17. 4 mL | 25. 8 mL |
| 2. 0.75 mL | 10. 0.5 tablet | 18. 18 or 20 mL | 26. 4 mL |
| 3. 1 tablet | 11. 19 mL or 21 mL | 19. 5 mL | 27. 1 mL |
| 4. 10 mL | 12. 10 mL | 20. 4.8 or 5 mL | 28. 2 tablets |
| 5. 1.5 mL | 13. 2 tablets | 21. 1.2 mL | 29. 1 mL |
| 6. 1 tablet | 14. 1 tablet | 22. 1 tablet | 30. 0.125 mL |
| 7. 2 tablets | 15. a. 7.5 mL  b. 2 vials | 23. 1 mL | |
| 8. 0.5 mL | 16. 7.5 mL | 24. 1.5 mL | |

# 6

## Chapter Six

# Reconstitution of Powdered Drugs

# Reconstitution of Powdered Drugs

### Introduction
Reconstitution of powdered drugs involves the addition of a diluent. This chapter explains: why drugs are stored in powdered form, how to reconstitute the drugs, how to select a diluent, the differentiation of IM vs IV dilution, proper labeling of the container after reconstitution of the drug, and storage after reconstitution.

### Why are Drugs Stored in Powdered Form?
Drugs are stored in powdered form to maintain stability and increase storage time. In dry powdered form the drug may have an expiration date of up to two years. This varies with each particular drug. The expiration date is printed on the label. When a diluent, such as normal saline or water, is added to the powdered drug the expiration date changes. After reconstitution the expiration date can range from hours to a month.

### How to Reconstitute a Drug in Powdered Form
Reconstitution of powdered drugs involves the addition of a sterile diluent, usually distilled water or normal saline, to a drug that is in the form of a powder. Under usual circumstances the reconstitution is done by the pharmacist. However, in many specialized areas such as the emergency room, the drugs are stored in the powdered form and need to be reconstituted.

The containers of the drugs or the package inserts will contain information on the manufacturer's directions for reconstitution, including the type of solution that should be used to reconstitute the drug. The most common solutions for reconstitution are sterile distilled water, sterile normal saline, or 5% dextrose and water. If the drug requires a special solution for dilution, it is usually supplied by the manufacturer of the drug and packaged with the drug.

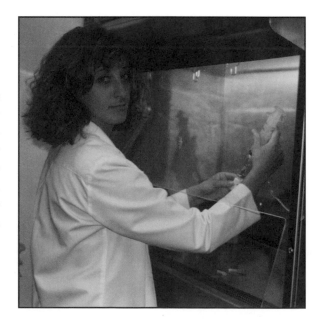

### Laminar Flow Hoods
The majority of drugs are reconstituted in the pharmacy under laminar flow hoods that filter the air. The hood filters out airborne contaminants. **Aseptic technique is required for preparation of parenteral drugs.** It is best to prepare medications away from the bedside in a clean aseptic environment. The photograph to the right shows an antibiotic being reconstituted under the laminar flow hood.

### Reconstitution of powdered drugs by the nurse
A nurse will occasionally reconstitute a powdered drug when it has to be done just before the drug is administered or in the nursing units such as the emergency room, operating room, recovery room, or intensive care where it is necessary to give the drug immediately.

## Terminology

**Diluent:** That which dilutes. The two most common diluents used are saline and water. The diluent that may be used can be determined by reading the drug label, package insert, or Physicians' Desk Reference. (PDR) The PDR states, for example, that penicillin G potassium is highly water soluble. It may be dissolved in small amounts of water for injection, or Sterile Isotonic Sodium Chloride for parenteral use.

**Solute:** The substance that is dissolved in the solution. Example: penicillin G in powdered form.

**Reconstitution:** Taking a drug in powdered form and restoring it to a drug in solution. For example, taking the powdered drug penicillin G and adding bacteriostatic water or saline to the vial to restore it to a solution.

**Solution:** A liquid containing a dissolved substance. For example, penicillin G with 23 mL of parenteral normal saline (NS) added to the vial is a solution with 200,000 units of penicillin per mL. Notice that the penicillin label tells how much diluent to add for different concentrations of the drug in solution.

### Labeling of drugs after reconstitution
Date and time the drug was prepared.
The initials of the person preparing the drug.
The concentration of the solution prepared.

**Note:** *If this information is not found on the label of a reconstituted drug, it must be discarded.*

### Storage of the drug after reconstituting
The label or package insert will state how to store the drug. For example, unused portions of penicillin G may be stored refrigerated for one week.

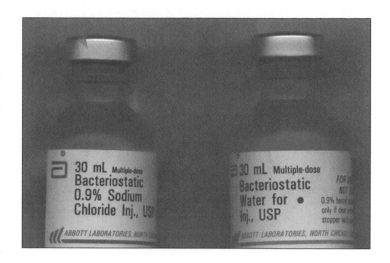

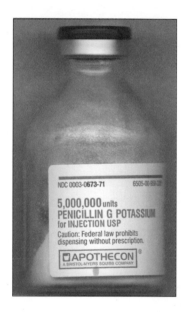

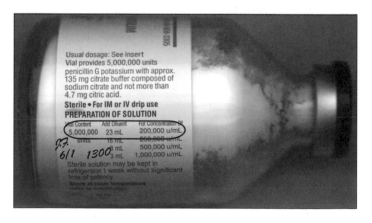

Read the label and answer the following questions.

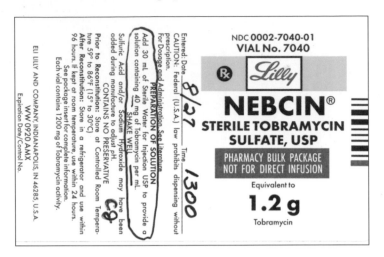

1. What type of diluent can be used?

   Answer: Sterile water for injection USP

2. How much diluent should be added to the vial?

   Answer: 30 mL

3. When was this drug reconstituted?

   Answer: 8/27

4. What are the initials of the person who prepared the drug?

   Answer: CJ

5. How long will this drug remain potent if refrigerated?

   Answer: 4 days

6. How long will this drug remain potent at room temperature?

   Answer: One day

7. What is the concentration of this drug per mL?

   Answer: 40 mg per mL

8. The doctor ordered 80 mg of tobramycin. What would you give?

   Answer: 2 mL

9. You found the drug in the patient's cubicle and today's date is 8/30.

   What would you do with this vial?

   Answer: Discard the drug because it is outdated after being stored at room temperature.

Remember to wash your hands before beginning preparation of any medication and use aseptic technique.

1. Read the Ampicillin label and selected part of package insert and then answer the questions below.

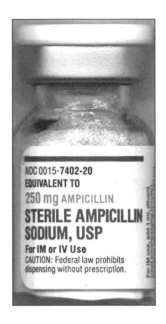

**DIRECTIONS FOR USE**

Use only freshly prepared solutions. Intramuscular and intravenous injections should be administered within one hour after preparation, since the potency may decrease significantly after this period.

**For Intramuscular Use**—Dissolve contents of a vial with the amount of Sterile Water for Injection, USP, or Bacteriostatic Water for Injection, USP, listed in the table below:

| NDC 0015 | Label Claim | Recommended Amount of Diluent | Withdrawable Volume | Concentration (in mg/mL) |
|----------|-------------|-------------------------------|---------------------|--------------------------|
| 7401-20 | 125 mg | 1.2 mL | 1.0 mL | 125 mg |
| 7402-20 | 250 mg | 1.0 mL | 1.0 mL | 250 mg |
| 7403-20 | 500 mg | 1.8 mL | 2.0 mL | 250 mg |
| 7404-20 | 1 gram | 3.5 mL | 4.0 mL | 250 mg |
| 7405-20 | 2 gram | 6.8 mL | 8.0 mL | 250 mg |

While Sterile Ampicillin Sodium, USP, 1 g and 2 g, are primarily for intravenous use, they may be administered intramuscularly when the 250 mg or 500 mg vials are unavailable. In such instances, dissolve in 3.5 or 6.8 mL Sterile Water for Injection, USP, or Bacteriostatic Water for Injection, USP, respectively. The resulting solution will provide a concentration of 250 mg per mL.

Sterile Ampicillin Sodium, USP, 125 mg, is intended primarily for pediatric use. It also serves as a convenient dosage form when small parenteral doses of the antibiotic are required.

**For Direct Intravenous Use**—Add 5 mL Sterile Water for Injection, USP, or Bacteriostatic Water for Injection, USP to the 125, 250, and 500 mg vials and administer slowly over a 3- to 5-minute period. Sterile Ampicillin Sodium, USP, 1 g or 2 g, may also be given by direct intravenous administration. Dissolve in 7.4 or 14.8 mL Sterile Water for Injection, USP, or Bacteriostatic Water for Injection, USP, respectively, and administer slowly over at least 10 to 15 minutes. CAUTION: More rapid administration may result in convulsive seizures.

**For Administration by Intravenous Drip**—Reconstitute as directed above (**For Direct Intravenous Use**) prior to diluting with Intravenous Solution. Stability studies on ampicillin sodium at several concentrations in various intravenous solutions indicate the drug will lose less than 10% activity at the temperatures noted for the time periods stated.

| Room Temperature (25° C) | | |
|--------------------------|---------------|------------------|
| Diluent | Concentrations | Stability Periods |
| Sterile Water for Injection | up to 30 mg/mL | 8 hours |
| Isotonic Sodium Chloride | up to 30 mg/mL | 8 hours |
| M/6 Sodium Lactate Solution | up to 30 mg/mL | 8 hours |
| 5% Dextrose in Water | 10 to 20 mg/mL | 2 hours |
| 5% Dextrose in Water | up to 2 mg/mL | 4 hours |
| 5% Dextrose in 0.45% NaCl | up to 2 mg/mL | 4 hours |
| 10% Invert Sugar in Water | up to 2 mg/mL | 4 hours |
| Lactated Ringer's Solution | up to 30 mg/mL | 8 hours |

| Refrigerated (4° C) | | |
|---------------------|---------------|------------------|
| Sterile Water for Injection | 30 mg/mL | 48 hours |
| Sterile Water for Injection | up to 20 mg/mL | 72 hours |
| Isotonic Sodium Chloride | 30 mg/mL | 48 hours |
| Isotonic Sodium Chloride | up to 20 mg/mL | 72 hours |
| Lactated Ringer's Solution | up to 30 mg/mL | 24 hours |
| M/6 Sodium Lactate Solution | up to 30 mg/mL | 8 hours |
| 5% Dextrose in Water | up to 20 mg/mL | 4 hours |
| 5% Dextrose in 0.45% NaCl | up to 10 mg/mL | 4 hours |
| 10% Invert Sugar | up to 20 mg/mL | 3 hours |

Only those solutions listed above should be used for the intravenous infusion of Sterile Ampicillin Sodium, USP. The concentrations should fall within the range specified. The drug concentration and the rate and volume of the infusion should be adjusted so that the total dose of ampicillin is administered before the drug loses its stability in the solution in use.

NDC 0015-7402-20
EQUIVALENT TO
250 mg AMPICILLIN
**STERILE AMPICILLIN SODIUM, USP**
For IM or IV Use
CAUTION: Federal law prohibits dispensing without prescription.

Prepare the Ampicillin for IV PB use to be added to 50 mL bag.

a. What types of diluent can be used? _____

b. How many mL should be added to the vial for administration by intravenous drip? _____

c. To give Ampicillin 250 mg how much would you draw up into a syringe? _____

d. If it was added to 50 mL bag of 5 % Dextrose in Water was used, how long will it maintain its stability refrigerated? _____

e. If added to 50 mL bag of 5 % Dextrose in Water, how long will it maintain its stability at room temperature? _____

f. Date and time this solution was prepared? _____

g. What are the initials of the person preparing this drug? _____

2. Read the label and prepare to give Librium 50 mg IM. Answer the questions below.

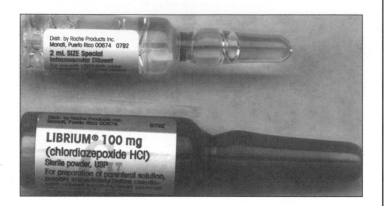

Preparation and Administration of Solutions: Package insert *Intramuscular:* Add 2 mL of *Special Intramuscular Diluent* to contents of 5-mL dry-filled amber ampul of Librium Sterile Powder (100 mg). Avoid excessive pressure in injecting this special diluent into the ampul containing powder since bubbles will form on the surface of the solution. Agitate gently until completely dissolved. Solution should be prepared immediately before administration. Any unused solution should be discarded. Deep intramuscular injection should be given slowly into the upper outer quadrant of the gluteus muscle.

Caution: Librium solution made with the Special Intramuscular Diluent should not be given intravenously because of the air bubbles which can form when the intramuscular diluent is added to the Librium powder. Do not use diluent solution if it is opalescent or hazy.

Librium is usually given IM. It can be given IV using 5 mL of sterile physiologic saline or sterile water for injection. Caution: Librium solution made with physiological saline or sterile water for injection should not be given intramuscularly because of pain on injection.

a. What type of diluent can be used? _____

b. How many mL should be added to the ampule? _____

c. To give Librium 50 mg, how many mL should be drawn up into the syringe?_____

d. After reconstitution, how long will this drug maintain its stability? _____

e. Can the left overdrug be used at a later time? _____

f. Is this diluent for intramuscular use only? _____

**Note:** *When a drug requires a special diluent, the manufacturer may package both the drug and the diluent. Librium is an example of this.*

3.  Read the Ancef label and answer the questions below.

| | |
|---|---|
| **equivalent to**<br>**1 gram** cefazolin<br>NDC 0007-3130-16<br><br>**ANCEF**®<br>**STERILE CEFAZOLIN**<br>**SODIUM (LYOPHILIZED)**<br><br>**25 Vials for Intramuscular**<br>**or Intravenous Use** | NSN 6505-01-262-9508<br>**Before reconstitution protect from light and store at**<br>**controlled room temperature (15° to 30°C; 59° to 86°F).**<br>**Usual Adult Dosage:** 250 mg to 1 gram every 6 to 8 hours.<br>See accompanying prescribing information.<br>For I.M. administration add 2.5 mL of Sterile Water for Injection.<br>SHAKE WELL. Withdraw entire contents. Provides an approxi-<br>mate volume of 3.0 mL (330 mg/mL). For I.V. administration see<br>accompanying prescribing information.<br>Reconstituted *Ancef* is stable for 24 hours at room temperature<br>or for 10 days if refrigerated (5°C or 41°F).<br>**SmithKline Beecham Pharmaceuticals**<br>Philadelphia, PA 19101      694115-N<br><br>K3130-16 |

Prepare Ancef for IM use.

a.  What type of diluent can be used?        _____

b.  How many mL should be added to the vial for IM use?        _____

c.  How many mg per mL?        _____

d.  To give Ancef 250 mg IM, how much would you draw into the syringe? _____

e.  When refrigerated, how long is Ancef stable?        _____

f.  When at room temperature, how long is Ancef stable?        _____

g.  Date and time the Ancef was prepared?        _____

h.  If this vial is labeled properly, can the unused portion be used again?        _____

4. Read the Chloromycetin label and answer the questions below.

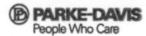

N 0071-4057-03

**Chloromycetin®**
**Sodium Succinate**
(Sterile Chloramphenicol
Sodium Succinate, USP)
Each vial delivers the equivalent of
**1 GRAM** chloramphenicol
**100 mg per mL** when reconstituted

Caution—Federal law prohibits
dispensing without prescription.

**PARKE-DAVIS**
People Who Care

Warning—Blood dyscrasias may be associated with the use of chloramphenicol. It is essential that adequate blood studies be made. See enclosed warnings and precautions.

For intravenous administration

Usual Adult Daily Dose—50 mg per kg. See package insert.

Contents have been freeze-dried in vial.

Store between 15° and 25°C (59° and 77°F).

Keep this and all drugs out of the reach of children.

To prepare a 10% (100 mg/mL) solution, add 10 mL of sterile aqueous diluent such as Sterile Water for Injection or 5% Dextrose Injection. When reconstituted as directed, 10 mL contains the equivalent of 1 gram chloramphenicol.

Solution may be kept at room temperature and should be used within 30 days. A cloudy solution should not be used.

**PARKE-DAVIS**
Div of Warner-Lambert Co ©1993
Morris Plains, NJ 07950 USA

a. What type of diluent can be used? _____

b. How many mL should be added to the vial? _____

c. How much would you draw into a syringe to give 500 mg? _____

d. Can Chloromycetin be kept at room temperature and maintain its stability? _____

e. Date and time the solution was prepared? _____

f. How many days will Chloromycetin maintain its stability after reconstitution?_____

g. Can Chloromycetin be used if the solution is cloudy? _____

5.  Read the Vancocin label and selected part of package insert, then answer the questions below.

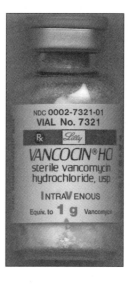

# VANCOCIN® HCl
## STERILE VANCOMYCIN HYDROCHLORIDE, USP
### INTRAVENOUS

Intermittent infusion is the recommended method of administration.
**PREPARATION AND STABILITY**

At the time of use, reconstitute by adding either 10 mL of Sterile Water for Injection to the 500-mg vial or 20 mL of Sterile Water for Injection to the 1-g vial of dry, sterile vancomycin powder. Vials reconstituted in this manner will give a solution of 50 mg/mL. FURTHER DILUTION IS REQUIRED.

After reconstitution, the vials may be stored in a refrigerator for 14 days without significant loss of potency. Reconstituted solutions containing 500 mg of vancomycin must be diluted with at least 100 mL of diluent. Reconstituted solutions containing 1 g of vancomycin must be diluted with at least 200 mL of diluent. The desired dose, diluted in this manner, should be administered by intermittent intravenous infusion over a period of at least 60 minutes.

*Compatibility With Intravenous Fluids*—Solutions that are diluted with 5% Dextrose Injection or 0.9% Sodium Chloride Injection may be stored in a refrigerator for 14 days without significant loss of potency. Solutions that are diluted with the following infusion fluids may be stored in a refrigerator for 96 hours:

 5% Dextrose Injection and 0.9% Sodium Chloride Injection, USP
 Lactated Ringer's Injection, USP
 Lactated Ringer's and 5% Dextrose Injection
 Normosol®-M and 5% Dextrose
 Isolyte® E
 Acetated Ringer's Injection
Vancomycin solution has a low pH that may cause chemical or physical instability when it is mixed with other compounds.

Prior to administration, parenteral drug products should be inspected visually for particulate matter and discoloration whenever solution or container permits.

a. What type of diluent can be used?  _____

b. How many mL should be added to the vial?  _____

c. How many mg are there per mL?  _____

d. How many mL should be drawn into the syringe to give 500 mg? _____

e. If diluted with normal saline and refrigerated, how many days
   will Vancocin maintain its stability?  _____

f. Does Vancocin need to be further diluted before it is given IV?  _____

g. Given IV PB, over what period of time should the piggyback run?_____

**Note:** *Vancocin is very irritating to the vein and therefore requires further dilution and a slower infusion rate than most intravenous piggybacks. This slower infusion rate helps to prevent phlebitis.*

6.  Read the Kefzol label and selected part of package insert then answer the questions below.

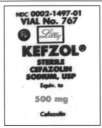

NDC 0002-1497-01
VIAL No. 767

*Lilly*

**KEFZOL®**
STERILE
CEFAZOLIN
SODIUM, USP
Equiv. to
**500 mg**
Cefazolin

### DOSAGE AND ADMINISTRATION

Kefzol may be administered intramuscularly or intravenously after reconstitution. Total daily dosages are the same for either route of administration.

*Intramuscular Administration*—Reconstitute as directed by Table 3 with 0.9% Sodium Chloride Injection, Sterile Water for Injection, or Bacteriostatic Water for Injection. Shake well until dissolved. Kefzol should be injected into a large muscle mass. Pain on injection is infrequent with Kefzol.

#### TABLE 3. DILUTION TABLE

| Vial Size | Diluent to Be Added | Approximate Available Volume | Approximate Average Concentration |
|---|---|---|---|
| 250 mg | 2 mL | 2 mL | 125 mg/mL |
| 500 mg | 2 mL | 2.2 mL | 225 mg/mL |
| 1 g* | 2.5 mL | 3 mL | 330 mg/mL |

*The 1-g vial should be reconstituted only with Sterile Water for Injection or Bacteriostatic Water for Injection.

*Intravenous Administration*—Kefzol may be administered by intravenous injection or by continuous or intermittent infusion.

Intermittent intravenous infusion: Kefzol can be administered along with primary intravenous fluid management programs in a volume control set or in a separate, secondary IV bottle. Reconstituted 500 mg or 1 g of Kefzol may be diluted in 50 to 100 mL of 1 of the following intravenous solutions: 0.9% Sodium Chloride Injection, 5% or 10% Dextrose Injection, 5% Dextrose in Lactated Ringer's Injection, 5% Dextrose and 0.9% Sodium Chloride Injection (also may be used with 5% Dextrose and 0.45% or 0.2% Sodium Chloride Injection), Lactated Ringer's Injection, 5% or 10% Invert Sugar in Sterile Water for Injection, Ringer's Injection, Normosol®-M in D5-W, Ionosol® B with Dextrose 5%, or Plasma-Lyte® with 5% Dextrose.

ADD-Vantage Vials of Kefzol are to be reconstituted *only* with 0.9% Sodium Chloride Injection or 5% Dextrose Injection in the 50-mL or 100-mL Flexible Diluent Containers.

Intravenous injection (Administer solution directly into vein or through tubing): Dilute the reconstituted 500 mg or 1 g of Kefzol in a minimum of 10 mL of Sterile Water for Injection. Inject solution slowly over 3 to 5 minutes. Do not inject in less than 3 minutes. (NOTE: ADD-VANTAGE VIALS ARE NOT TO BE USED IN THIS MANNER.)

*Dosage*—The usual adult dosages are given in Table 4.

#### TABLE 4. USUAL ADULT DOSAGE

| Type of Infection | Dose | Frequency |
|---|---|---|
| Pneumococcal pneumonia | 500 mg | q12h |
| Mild infections caused by susceptible gram-positive cocci | 250 to 500 mg | q8h |
| Acute uncomplicated urinary tract infections | 1 g | q12h |
| Moderate to severe infections | 500 mg to 1 g | q6 to 8h |
| Severe, life-threatening infections (eg, endocarditis, and septicemia)* | 1 g to 1.5 g | q6h |

*In rare instances, doses up to 12 g of cefazolin per day have been used.

a. What diluents can be used for the 500 mg vial for IM use? _____

b. How many mL should be added to the vial? _____

c. How many mg are there per 2.2 mL? _____

d. To administer 300 mg, how many mL should be drawn into the syringe? _____

e. List the solutions with which Kefzol can be further diluted? _____

_____

f. What are the three ways Kefzol may be given intravenously? _____

_____

_____

Answers: Chapter 6, 1-6

1.  a.  Sterile water for injection, isotonic sodium chloride, D5W, D5 0.45NS, LR, 10% invert sugar, bacteriostatic water for injection.
    b.  5 mL
    c.  5 mL or all of it
    d.  4 hours
    e.  2 hours
    f.  Today's date and time should be written on the piggyback
    g.  Your initials should be written on the piggyback
2.  a.  The special diluent provided by the manufacturer
    b.  2 mL
    c.  1 mL
    d.  Just a short time, must be mixed just prior to administration
    e.  No. Discard any unused portions
    f.  Yes. This diluent is for intramuscular use only. Librium is usually given IM, but if it is necessary to give it IV, sterile water or physiologic saline for injection may be used.
3.  a.  Sterile water for injection
    b.  2.5 mL
    c.  330 mg per mL
    d.  0.76 mL
    e.  10 days
    f.  24 hours
    g.  Today's date and time
    h.  Yes
4.  a.  Sterile water for injection, D5W
    b.  10 mL
    c.  5 mL
    d.  Yes
    e.  Today's date and time
    f.  30 days
    g.  No
5.  a.  Sterile water for injection, 5% Dextrose Injection, 0.9% Sodium Chloride Injection, Lactated Ringer's Injection, Normosol M, Isolyte E, and acetated Ringer's Injection.
    b.  20 mL
    c.  50 mg/mL
    d.  10 mL
    e.  14 days
    f.  Yes in 100 mL for 500mg
    g.  Over 60 minutes
6.  a.  Sterile Water for Injection or Bacteriostatic Water for Injection& 0.9 % Sodium Chloride Injection
    b.  2 mL
    c.  225 mg/mL
    d.  1.3 mL
    e.  0.9 Sodium Chloride Injection, 5% or 10% Dextrose Injection, 5% Dextrose and Ringers Lactate, 5% Dextrose and Normal Saline, 5% Dextrose and 0.45% Normal Saline, 5% Dextrose and 0.2% Normal Saline, Lactated Ringer's, Ringer's, Normosol M, Ionosol B with 5% Dextrose and Plasma Lyte with 5% Dextrose.
    f.  Kefzol can be further diluted with any of the above solutions. 1. It can be given with a soluset along with the primary IV fluids. 2. It can be given separately as an IV PB 3. It can be further diluted in 10 mL of Sterile Water for Injection and given slowly over 3-5 minutes.

# Notes

# 7

## Chapter Seven

## Pediatric Drug Calculation

Author:   Ginger Kee, Ed D., R. N.
Associate Professor of Clinical Nursing
University of Texas, Houston

# Pediatric Drug Calculation

## Introduction

After completing this chapter you will be able to: explain the nurse's responsibility in administering medications to children, calculate safe dosages for children, determine safe dosages for children, determine the amount of a medication to prepare, determine safe IV dilution and rate, and calculate a child's body surface area based on a Nomogram Chart. Each concept that is presented will be followed by practice problems.

## Children's Dosages

Calculation of medications for children is done in the same manner as adult calculations except that the dosage is individualized according to the child's age, weight and/or body surface area. Children's dosages are smaller than adult dosages due to their size, body surface area, metabolism, and the ability to absorb and excrete medications. The difference between 9 mL and 0.9 mL is 10 times the dosage. Nurses have to be particularly alert when computing and administering medications to infants and children. Frequently, the dosage range varies with the following ages:

| | |
|---|---|
| Neonate | 0-1 month |
| Infant | 1 month - 12 months |
| Child | 1 year - 12 years |

There is little margin for error when preparing medications for children.

Since many children have difficulty swallowing tablets, most oral medications are in liquid or suspension form. Oral liquid measurements need to be exact and are measured in syringes, measuring spoons, or medication cups.

## Nursing Responsibilities

Some medications can be given by only one route (po, IV or IM). Nurses must check the ordered medication route to assure that the form of the medication is consistent with the order. The nurse's responsibility is to assure: (a) the medication can be administered by the route ordered, (b) the medication is in the correct form for the route ordered, and (c) the volume that is available can be safely administered by the route ordered.

Most nurses are not responsible for ordering the amount of medication. They *are* responsible for determining that the dosage ordered falls within a safe range for a particular child. The safe range can be determined by referring to a medication handbook for children or by calling the pharmacist.

## Safe Range

The safe range of dosage has a minimum and maximum dosage. A dosage that exceeds the maximum may cause serious toxic reactions and side effects. When the dosage ordered is less than the minimum amount, therapeutic effects of the drug may not occur.

## Nurse's Legal Responsibility

When the dosage ordered is outside the safe range or there are some questions regarding the preparation or route of administration, the nurse should follow these procedures before notifying the physician. First, the nurse should check the order for accuracy. Second, the history and physical condition of the patient should be taken into account to determine if there is a reasonable explanation for the discrepancy. Third, the nurse should check the serum level if applicable. Fourth, the nurse should check with the pharmacy to determine if the information is accurate. If there is still a concern, the nurse should notify the physician before proceeding. Remember, the nurse is legally liable for any medication administered.

## Double Check

Most hospitals have regulations requiring specific medications to be double-checked by another licensed individual before being administered. Such a policy is especially important in giving medications to children because the nurse frequently administers very small amounts and precision is critical. Medications which frequently require such precautions are **digoxin, heparin, insulin, epinephrine, narcotics, and sedatives**. Another licensed person should check calculations and amounts on those medications whether or not it is mandated.

| DOUBLE CHECK CALCULATIONS | |
|---|---|
| digoxin | narcotics |
| heparin | sedatives |
| insulin | epinephrine |

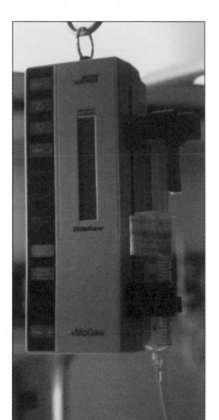

## Syringe Pump

Most of the IV PBs are now given with syringe pumps. They are safer, and more cost effective then using the soluset. Many facilities have or are in the process of switching to this method of delivering IV drugs.

## Fluids with IV Meds

Fluid overload can occur easily in infants and children with disastrous results. IV fluids are supplied in 250, 500 and 1000 mL amounts. The soluset may still be used to prevent fluid overload for an infant or child.

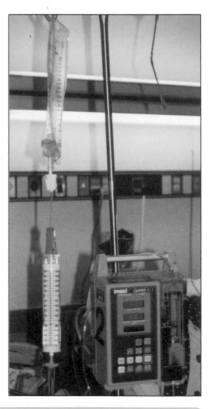

# Rounding Off Children's Dosages and Weights

Generally, in the care of children, calculations are carried out to the nearest thousandth (three digits to the right of the decimal - 0.000) and rounded to the nearest hundredth (two digits to the right of the decimal - 0.00). However, when the medication is more than 1 mL, calculate to the nearest hundredth and round to the nearest tenth.

## 1 mL or more
**If the dosage is 1 mL or more, calculate to the hundredth place** (0.00) and round to the nearest tenth (0.0)

## Round to tenth
To round off to the nearest tenth when the number in the hundredth place is less than 5, the number in the hundredth place is dropped and the number in the tenth place remains the same.

> 6.63
> 6.6 (the 3 is dropped, the 6 remains unchanged, because the 3 is less than 5)

To round off to the nearest tenth when the number in the hundredth place is equal to or greater than 5, the number in the hundredth place is dropped but the number in the tenth place is increased by 1.

> 6.68
> 6.7 (the 8 is dropped and the 6 is increased by 1, because 8 is greater than 5)

## Less than 1 mL
If the dosage is less than 1 mL, calculate thousandths (0.000) and round off to the nearest hundredth (0.00). A tuberculin syringe is used to measure the dosage in hundredths.

## Round to hundredth
To round off to the nearest hundredth when the number in the thousandth place is less than 5, the number in the thousandth place is dropped, and the number in the hundredth place remains the same.

> 0.932
> 0.93 (the 2 is dropped, the 3 remains unchanged, because it is less than 5)

To round off to the nearest hundredths when the number is in the thousandth place is equal to or greater than 5, the number in the thousandths place is dropped and the number in the hundredth place is increased by 1

> 0.937
> 0.94 (the 7 is dropped and the 3 is increased by one, because 7 is greater than 5)

## Rounding Off Children's Dosages

Round off each of the following problems to the nearest tenth or hundredth according to the appropriate dosage in milliliters.

1.  0.135  _____
2.  1.756  _____
3.  3.567  _____
4.  0.257  _____
5.  0.753  _____

6.  4.632  _____
7.  0.917  _____
8.  9.148  _____
9.  3.795  _____
10. 0.112  _____

Answers: Practice Problems chapter 7, 1-10

| | | | |
|---|---|---|---|
| 1. 0.14 | 4. 0.26 | 7. 0.92 | 10. 0.11 |
| 2. 1.8 | 5. 0.75 | 8. 9.1 | |
| 3. 3.6 | 6. 4.6 | 9. 3.8 | |

# Children's Dosage

Before drawing up a medication dosage for a newborn, infant, or child, you should assure that the prescribed drug is within a safe range. Safe ranges most frequently are determined by age or weight.

| Example by Age Acetaminophen | |
|---|---|
| 0-3 mo | 40 mg/dosage |
| 4-11 mo | 80 mg/dosage |
| 12-24 mo | 120 mg/dosage |
| 2-3 yrs | 160 mg/dosage |
| 4-5 yrs | 240 mg/dosage |
| 6-8 yrs | 320 mg/dosage |
| 9-10 yrs | 400 mg/dosage |
| 11-12 yrs | 480 mg/dosage |

**Example by weight Acetaminophen**

10 - 15 mg/kg/dosage

All systemic medications should have safe dosage calculated whether they are given orally, IM, SC, or IV. The following sample and practice problems have the medication safe ranges calculated by weight. Safe range could be mg/kg/dosage (most prn meds) or mg/kg/24 hours (most other medications). Review the sample problems on how to calculate the safe dosage range and amount for children.

You must be able to convert pounds to kilograms before the safe dosage can be calculated.

When converting pounds (lbs) to kilograms (kg), calculate to thousandths and round to nearest hundredth.

# Convert Pounds to Kilograms and Round to Nearest Hundredth.

Infant's weight:     10 lbs, 12 oz

1.  **Convert ounces to pounds**

    16 oz = 1 lb

    Set up ratio and proportion

    $$\frac{16 \text{ oz}}{1 \text{ lb}} = \frac{12 \text{ oz}}{X \text{ lb}}$$

    16 X = 12

    $$X = \frac{12}{16} = \frac{3}{4} = 0.75$$

    X = 0.75 lbs

    Answer: The infant weighs 10.75 lbs

2.  **Convert pounds to kilograms**

    2.2 lbs = 1 kg

    $$\frac{2.2 \text{ lbs}}{1 \text{ kg}} = \frac{10.75 \text{ lbs}}{X \text{ kg}}$$

    2.2 X = 10.75

    $$X = \frac{10.75}{2.2}$$

    X = 4.886 kg

3.  **Round off to nearest hundredth**          **Simplified formula**

    4.886 = 4.89 kg                              $$kg = \frac{lbs}{2.2}$$

    Answer: infant weighs 4.89 kg

# Safe Dosage Calculation Problem

■ *Physician orders Ilosone (erythromycin) 62.5 mg, po q6h for an 11 lb, 4 oz infant*

## A. What is infant's weight in kg?

4 oz = 4/16 or 1/4 or 0.25 lbs

Convert ounces to pounds          16 oz = 1 lb

2.2 lbs = 1 kg

$$\frac{2.2 \text{ lbs}}{1 \text{ kg}} = \frac{11.25 \text{ lbs}}{X \text{ kg}}$$

$$2.2X = 11.25$$

$$X = \frac{11.25}{2.2}$$

$$X = 5.113 \text{ or } 5.11 \text{ kg}$$

Answer: The infant weighs 5.11 kg.

## B. What is the safe 24 hour dosage range for this infant?

Consult a reference for the safe dosage range.
According to *The Harriet Lane Handbook,* the safe dosage range for erythromycin is 30-50 mg/kg/24 hours divided every 6 hrs.

Calculate the safe 24 hour dosage range for this particular infant.

5.11 kg x 30 = 153.3 mg

5.11 kg x 50 = 255.5 mg

Answer: The safe 24 hour dosage range is 153.3 - 255.5 mg/24 hrs

## C. What is the safe single dosage range?

The safe single dosage range is the safe 24 hour range divided by the frequency ordered.
Calculate the safe dosage range for each 6 hour dosage for this infant. A medication given every 6 hours is given 4 times per day (24 hours divided by 6)

$$\frac{153.3}{4} = 38.325 \text{ mg (38.33 with rounding)}$$

$$\frac{255.5}{4} = 63.875 \text{ mg (63.88 with rounding)}$$

Answer: Safe dosage range is 38.32-63.88 mg every 6 hours

D.  **Is the ordered dosage within the safe range?**

>   Answer: Yes. The ordered dosage of 62.5 mg q6h falls between 38.33 and 63.88 mg.
>   It is within the safe dosage range.

E.  **How many mg should be given per dosage?**

>   Answer: 62.5 mg

**Note:** *Always give what is ordered unless it is unsafe. You may not change the amount of medication ordered without a physician's order. You should complete the appropriate checks and notify the physician if concerns persist.*

F.  **What route should the ordered medication be given?**

>   Answer: po

**Note:** *Always administer medications by route ordered. If there is a concern, you should complete the appropriate checks and then notify the physician that the route is questionable. You may not change the route without a physician's order.*

G.  **How many mL of medication should be drawn up?**

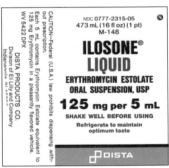

Determine the number of mL to be prepared based on the label.

>   Set up ratio and proportion

$$\frac{125 \text{ mg}}{5 \text{ mL}} = \frac{62.5 \text{ mg}}{X \text{ mL}}$$

$$125\,X = 312.5$$

$$X = \frac{312.5}{125}$$

$$X = 2.5 \text{ mL}$$

Answer: 2.5 mL of erythromycin 125 mg/5 mL should be prepared to deliver 62.5 mg as ordered.

**H. How many teaspoons would equal the ordered amount?**

Determine the number of teaspoons

You need to know how to convert to household measures

Set up ratio and proportion

$$\frac{5 \text{ mL}}{1 \text{ tsp}} = \frac{2.5 \text{ mL}}{X \text{ tsp}}$$

$$5 X = 2.5$$

$$X = \frac{2.5}{5}$$

$$X = 0.5 \text{ or } \frac{1}{2} \text{ tsp}$$

**Simplified formula**

$$\text{Teaspoons} = \frac{\text{mL}}{5}$$

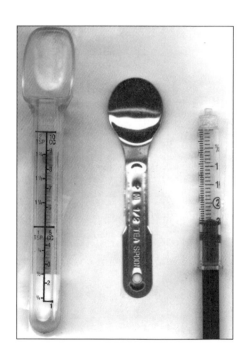

Answer: ½ teaspoon equals the ordered amount.

**I. Would the teaspoon measurement be practical?**

Answer: Yes

**Note:** *Sometimes the dosage can not be safely measured in household device measures. When that is the case, instruct someone in the family on how to draw up the medication into a syringe and send the syringes home with that person. One-half teaspoon can be measured with all of the devices pictured.*

11. The physician orders Proventil (albuterol) 0.5 mg, po, q8h. The infant weighs 11 lbs, 4 oz. *The Harriet Lane Handbook* states that the safe dosage for albuterol is 0.3 mg/kg/24 hours divided every 8 hours.

A. What is the infant's weight in kg?  _____

B. What is the safe 24 hour dosage range for this infant?  _____

C. What is the safe single dosage range?  _____

D. Is the dosage ordered within the safe range?  _____

E. How many mg should you give per dosage?  _____

F. What route should the medication be given?  _____

G. How many mL of medication should be prepared?  _____

H. How many teaspoons equal the ordered amount?  _____

I. Is the teaspoon measurement practical?  _____

> NDC 0093-0661-16
> 6505-01-256-4997
> ALBUTEROL
> SULFATE
> Syrup
> 2 mg/5 mL

12. The physician orders Ferrous Sulfate (iron preparation), 9 mg, po, tid. The child weighs 14 lbs, 8 oz. *The Harriet Lane Handbook* states that the safe dosage for iron (Fe) is 3 - 6 mg of elemental Fe/kg/24 hours divided tid.

A. What is the child's weight in kg?  _____

B. What is the safe 24 hour dosage range for this child?  _____

C. What is the safe single dosage range?  _____

D. Is the dosage ordered within the safe range?  _____

E. How many mg should you give per dosage?  _____

F. By what route should the medication be given?  _____

G. How many mL of medication should be prepared?  _____

H. Could a dropper that comes with Ferrous Sulfate be used?_____

I. Would a TB syringe measurement be practical?  _____

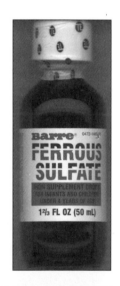

> DAILY USAGE: 0.6 mL daily.
> 0.6 mL supplies 15 mg of elemental iron—
> 100% of the U.S. Recommended Daily Allowance (U.S. RDA) for infants and 150% of the U.S. RDA for children under 4 years of age.
>
> May be dropped directly into mouth with dropper or mixed with water, fruit juice, cereal or other food.
>
> EACH 0.6 mL CONTAINS:
> Iron . . . . . . . . . . . . . . . . . . . . . . . 15 mg
> (as Ferrous Sulfate)

13. The physician orders Pediaprofen (ibuprofen) 20 mg po, q6h prn for temperature above 102. The infant is 1 ½ month old and weighs 9 lbs. *The Harriet Lane Handbook* states that the safe dosage for ibuprofen is 20-40 mg/kg/24 hours divided every 6 hours.

A.  What is the infant's weight in kg?                                    _____

B.  What is the safe 24 hour dosage range for this infant?   _____

C.  What is the safe single dosage range?                          _____

D.  Is the dosage ordered within the safe range?               _____

E.  How many mg should you give per dosage?                   _____

F.  By what route should the medication be given?             _____

G.  How many mL of medication should be prepared?        _____

H.  How many teaspoons equal the ordered amount?         _____

I.  Is the teaspoon measurement practical?                         _____

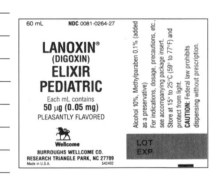

14. The physician orders Lanoxin (digoxin) 18 mcg, po, bid. The infant is 2 months old and weighs 7 lbs, 4 oz. *The Harriet Lane Handbook* states that the safe dosage for digoxin in children under 2 years of age is 10-12 mcg/kg/24 hours divided bid.

A.  What is the infants weight in kg?                                    _____

B.  What is the safe 24 hour dosage range for this infant?   _____

C.  What is the safe single dosage range?                          _____

D.  Is the dosage ordered within safe and therapeutic range?   _____

E.  How many mcg should you give per dosage?                 _____

F.  By what route should the ordered medication be given?   _____

G.  How many mL of medication should be prepared?        _____

H.  How many teaspoons equal the ordered amount?         _____

**Not appropriate:** *Digoxin should not be given in a teaspoon measure. It should be given in exact measurement. If the dropper in the digoxin bottle is exact, the family can use the dropper. If it is not exact, teach the family how to draw up digoxin into the syringe.*

15. The physician orders Dilantin (phenytoin) 40 mg po, q8h. The child is a 26 month old who weighs 27 lbs, 12 oz. *The Harriet Lane Handbook* states that the safe dosage for phenytoin as a seizure medication is 8 - 10 mg/kg/24 hours divided every 8 - 12 hours for children 6 months to 3 yrs.

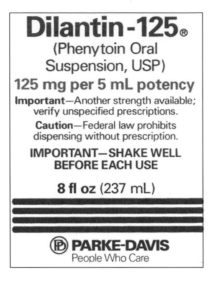

A.   What is the child's weight in kg?                                    _____

B.   What is the safe 24 hour dosage range for this child?          _____

C.   What is the safe single dosage range?                              _____

D.   Is the dosage ordered within the safe and therapeutic range? _____

E.   How many mg should you give per dosage?                       _____

F.   By what route should the medication be given?                  _____

G.   How many mL of medication should be prepared?               _____

H.   How many teaspoons equal the ordered amount?               _____

I.   Is the teaspoon measurement practical?                          _____

16. The physician orders prednisone 150 mg, po, bid. The child weighs 20 lbs, 8oz. *The Harriet Lane Hand-book* states that for an acute asthmatic attack, the safe dosage for oral prednisone is 0.5 - 40 mg/kg/24.

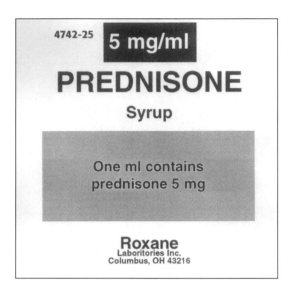

A. What is the child's weight in kg? _____

B. What is the safe 24 hour dosage range for this child? _____

C. What is the safe single dosage range? _____

D. Is the dosage ordered within the safe and therapeutic range? _____

E. How many mg should you give per dosage? _____

F. By what route should the ordered medication be given? _____

G. How many mL of medication should be prepared? _____

H. How many teaspoons equal the ordered amount? _____

I. Is the teaspoon measurement practical? _____

17. The physician orders Ceclor (cefaclor) 180 mg, po, q8h. The infant weighs 10 lbs. *The Harriet Lane Handbook* states that the safe dosage for cefaclor is 40 mg/kg/24 hours divided every 8 hours.

A.  What is the infant's weight in kg? _____

B.  What is the safe 24 hour dosage range for this infant? _____

C.  What is the safe single dosage range? _____

D.  Is the dosage ordered within the safe and therapeutic range? _____

E.  How many mg should you give per dosage? _____

F.  By what route should the medication be given? _____

G.  How many mL of medication should be prepared? _____

H.  How many teaspoons equal the ordered amount? _____

I.  Is the teaspoon measurement practical? _____

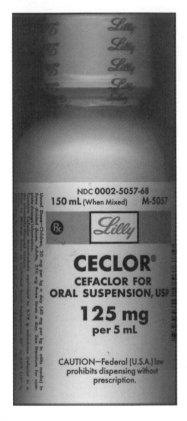

NDC 0002-5057-68
150 mL (When Mixed)   M-5057

℞   *Lilly*

**CECLOR®**
CEFACLOR FOR
ORAL SUSPENSION, USP

**125 mg**
per 5 mL

CAUTION—Federal (U.S.A.) law
prohibits dispensing without
prescription.

18. The physician orders Luminal (phenobarbital or PBS) 45 mg, po, bid. The child is 3 years old with seizures and weighs 35 lbs. *The Harriet Lane Handbook* states that for children 1 - 5 years of age, the safe dosage for phenobarbital for seizures is 6 -8 mg/kg/24 hours given everyday or bid.

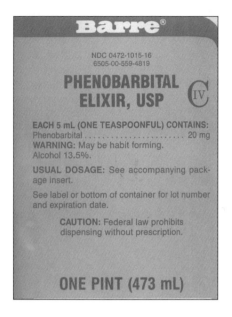

A. What is the child's weight in kg?  _____

B. What is the safe 24 hour dosage range for this child?  _____

C. What is the safe single dosage range?  _____

D. Is the dosage ordered within the safe range?  _____

E. How many mg should you give per dosage?  _____

F. By what route should the medication be given?  _____

G. How many mL of medication should be prepared?  _____

H. How many teaspoons equal the ordered amount?  _____

I. Is the teaspoon measurement practical?  _____

19. The physician has ordered Proventil (albuterol), 1.2 mg, po, every 8 hours. The child weighs 27 lbs. *The Harriet Lane Handbook* states that the safe dosage for albuterol is 0.3 mg/kg/24 hours divided every 8 hours.

   A.  What is the child's weight in kg?  _____

   B.  What is the safe 24 hour dosage range for this child?  _____

   C.  What is the safe single dosage range?  _____

   D.  Is the dosage ordered within the safe and therapeutic range? _____

   E.  How many mg should you give per dosage?  _____

   F.  By what route should the ordered medication be given?  _____

   G.  How many mL of medication should be prepared?  _____

   H.  How many teaspoons equal the ordered amount?  _____

   I.  Is the teaspoon measurement practical?  _____

   NDC 0093-0661-16
   6505-01-256-4997
   **ALBUTEROL SULFATE** Syrup
   **2 mg/5 mL**

20. The physician orders Tylenol (acetaminophen), 240 mg po, q4h prn for temp above 101. The child weighs 60 lbs. *The Harriet Lane Handbook* states that the safe dosage for acetaminophen is 10 - 15mg/kg/dosage every 4 hours, PRN

   A.  What is the child's weight in kg?  _____

   B.  What is the safe 24 hour dosage range for this child?  _____

   **Not appropriate:** *Medication is PRN and safe dose is calculated per dose not per 24 hours.*

   C.  What is the safe single dosage range?  _____

   D.  Is the dosage ordered within the safe and therapeutic range?  _____

   E.  How many mg should you give per dosage?  _____

   F.  By what route should the medication be given?  _____

   G.  How many mL of medication should be prepared?  _____

   H.  How many teaspoons equal the ordered amount?  _____

   I.  Is the teaspoon measurement practical?  _____

   NDC 0054-3010-50   120 mL
   **ACETAMINOPHEN**
   **(Cherry)**
   **Oral Solution USP**
   **160 mg per 5 mL**
   ANALGESIC-ANTIPYRETIC
   Alcohol-Free
   Each 5 mL (teaspoonful) contains:
   Acetaminophen 160 mg
   The seal of this package bears our
   name, Roxane. If this seal is broken or
   our name does not appear, do not use.
   Store at Controlled Room
   Temperature 15°-30°C (59°-86°F)
   4078000 033
   © RLI, 1993.   **Roxane** Laboratories, Inc.
   Columbus, Ohio 43216   120 mL (4.06 fl oz)

See Chapter Eight for more information about intravenous infusion rates.

■ The physician orders Kefurox (cefuroxime) 350 mg IV q8h. The 10 month old infant weighs 16 lbs, 8 oz. The nurse adds 3 mL of diluent to the vial.

### A.  What is the infant's weight in kg?

Convert lbs to kg  The infant weighs 16.5 lbs.

$$2.2 \text{ lbs} = 1 \text{ kg}$$

$$\frac{2.2 \text{ lbs}}{1 \text{ kg}} = \frac{16.5 \text{ lbs}}{X \text{ kg}}$$

Note:  8 oz = 8/16 or 1/2 or 0.5 lbs.

$$2.2 \text{ X} = 16.5$$

$$X = \frac{16.5}{2.2}$$

$$X = 7.5 \text{ kg}$$

Answer:  The infant weighs 7.5 kg

### B.  What is the safe 24 hour dosage range for this infant?

Consult a reference for the safe dosage range. *The Harriet Lane Handbook* states that the safe dosage for cefuroxime in infants and children is 75 - 150 mg/kg/24 hours divided every 8 hours.

Calculate the safe dosage range for 24 hours

$$7.5 \text{ kg} \times 75 = 562.5 \text{ mg}$$

$$7.5 \text{ kg} \times 150 \text{ mg} = 1125 \text{ mg}$$

Answer: Safe 24 hour dosage range is 562.5 - 1125 mg/24 hours

### C.  What is the safe single dosage range?

Calculate the safe dosage range for each 8 hour dosage

$$\frac{562.5}{3} = 187.5 \text{ mg}$$

$$\frac{1125}{3} = 375 \text{ mg}$$

Answer: Safe dosage range is 187.5 - 375 mg every 8 hours

### D. Is the ordered dosage within the safe range?

Answer: Yes:    The ordered dosage of 350 mg q8h falls between
187.5 - 375 mg and is within the safe dosage range

### E. How many mg should you give per dosage?

Answer : 350 mg

**Note:** *Give what is ordered unless it is unsafe. You may not change the amount of medication ordered without a physician's order.*

### F. What route should the ordered medication be given?

Answer: IV

**Note:** *Administer medications by route ordered. If there is a concern, you must make the appropriate checks. You may not change the route without a physician's order.*

**Note:** *It is essential that you know by which route a medication may be safely given. Also, you need to assure that the form of the medication that is available may be given by the route ordered.*

### G. How many mL of medication should be drawn up for IM use to be further diluted for IV Use?

**Note:** *Some medications come in dry form (cefuroxime, 750 mg vial) and some come in liquid form (gentamycin, 80 mg/mL).*

**Liquid Form:** The number of mg/mL will be indicated on the vial or ampule with the liquid form of medication.

**Dry form:** Before preparing the medication, it will have to be reconstituted. The vial will usually indicate the number of mL which are required to reconstitute the dry form into liquid form. It may or may not indicate the number of mg/mL the reconstitution yields. Due to displacement, the amount of liquid in the vial is usually greater than the amount of diluent the nurse added to the vial. If there is no indication of how many mg/mL the reconstitute yields, the nurse is required to measure the entire contents of the vial with a syringe to determine the resulting volume and strength of the medication. Once the volume and strength of the medication is determined, you can calculate the amount of medication which will be needed to deliver the ordered dosage.

Sample problems will include both liquid and powder forms of medications.

**Note:** *This label indicates that you can choose to dilute the medication in either 3.6 or 9 mL. Each amount will yield a different concentration. It is crucial that you know what the concentration is before determining how many mL would equal the ordered dosage. The nurse diluted the medication in 3.6 mL which yields 220 mg/mL, according to the package insert.*

**Note:** *Dry forms of medications are frequently diluted for IM use. Further dilution for IV use may be required. Medication examples will be diluted for IM use and further diluted for IV administration as indicated.*

Set up ratio and proportion

$$\frac{220 \text{ mg}}{1 \text{ mL}} = \frac{350 \text{ mg}}{X \text{ mL}}$$

220 X = 350

$$X = \frac{350}{220}$$

X = 1.59 or 1.6 with rounding

Answer: The nurse should draw up 1.6 mL of cefuroxime to have 350 mg.

**Note:** *If the medication is to be given IM, the nurse should give 1.6 mL. Since it is being given IV, the appropriate dilution and rate will need to be calculated.*

**Note:** *Before giving an IM injection you need to evaluate the size of the child and muscle mass. In infants and small children, the maximum amount of medication which may be given IM is 1 mL. This is in contrast to the 3 mL volume which may be given to adults. You will be asked to calculate the volume which is required to administer the medication IM. Frequently, the volume of medication to deliver the ordered dosage IM safely would require too many injections to be practical.*

## H. What volume of fluid would be needed for maximum IV concentration?

Determine the maximum concentration of cefuroxime to safely administer this medication IV.

**Note:** *There are established concentrations and rate of IV medications administration. The concentration and rate of administration must be followed to safely give IV medications. The drug is initially drawn up for IM use and then appropriately diluted for IV use.*

Consult a reference or pharmacist for recommended IV concentration and rate of administration. *The Pediatric Dosage Handbook* states cefuroxime intermittent infusion should be administered over 15 -30 minutes at a concentration of 30 mg/mL.

Determine the maximum concentration to safely give cefuroxime 350 mg.

$$\frac{30 \text{ mg}}{1 \text{ mL}} = \frac{350 \text{ mg}}{X \text{ mL}}$$

$$30 X = 350$$

$$X = \frac{350 \text{ mg}}{30}$$

$$X = 11.7 \text{ mL}$$

Answer: Dilute the 1.6 mL of cefuroxime to get a total volume of 11.7 mL

## I.   What rate should the medication be delivered IV?

Determine the IV rate to safely give 350 mg of cefuroxime at 9 AM.

Set up IV drip formula

**Note:** *All children's IV's should be on micro drip or machine. These deliver 60 gtts per cc or 60 mL/h thus the drip factor should be 60.*

$$\frac{\text{Number of mL x drip factor}}{\text{Number of minutes}}$$

$$\frac{11.7 \text{ mL x } 600 \text{ mL}}{15 \text{ min}} = \frac{702}{15} = 46.8 \text{ mL/hr or gtts/min}$$

To

$$\frac{11.7 \text{ mL x } 600}{30 \text{ min}} = \frac{702}{30} = 23.4 \text{ mL/hr or gtts/min}$$

Answer: The 11.7 mL of diluted cefuroxime can be given at a rate of 23.4 - 46.8 mL/hr or gtts/min

**Note:** *The stated volume may seem like a small amount to give IV. This is not unusual in the care of small infants and children. There is equipment which can deliver IV fluids in these volumes. The size of the child, physiologic status, characteristics of the drug, and hospital policy will determine whether this amount will be given or if it will be further diluted. Unless indicated otherwise, this chapter will use the most concentrated of the usual concentration (most mg/mL) for calculating IV dilution. Usual dilution is frequently less concentrated than maximum concentrtion indicated. IV medications should not be given in a volume less than maximum indicates. Increasing the volume of diluent is acceptable practice.*

The letter by each of the answers in the sample problem corresponds to the questions asked in each of the practice problems. This should help you refer to the example in answering the questions.

21. The physician orders gentamycin 25 mg IV q8h. The infant weighs 22 lbs, 12 oz. According to *The Harriet Lane Handbook*, the safe dosage for gentamicin is 6 - 7.5 mg/kg/24 hrs divided every 8 hrs. *The Pediatric Dosage Handbook* states that the safe IV concentration for gentamicin should not exceed 10 mg/mL and should be given over 30 minutes.

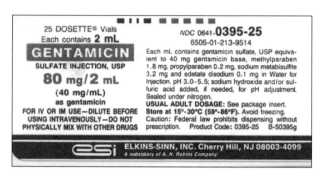

A. What is the infant's weight in kg? _____

B. What is the safe 24 hour dosage range. _____

C. What is the safe single dosage range? _____

D Is this dosage ordered within the safe and therapeutic range? _____

E. How many mg should be given per dosage? _____

F. By what route should the ordered medication be given? _____

G. How many mL of medication should be prepared for IM use

which will then be diluted for IV use? _____

H. What volume of fluid is needed for maximum IV concentration? _____

I. What rate should the medication be delivered IV? _____

22. The physician orders morphine sulfate (MS), 5 mg IV q2h prn for pain. The child weighs 55 lbs. According to *The Harriet Lane Handbook,* the safe dosage for morphine is 0.1 - 0.2 mg/kg/dosage every 2 - 4 hrs. *The Pediatric Dosage Handbook* states that morphine can be given IV push over at least 5 minutes or by intermittent infusion over 15-30 minutes at a concentration of 0.5 - 5 mg/mL. The nurse decides to give the morphine by IV push.

A. What is the child's weight in kg?   _____

B. What is the safe 24 hour dosage range?   _____

**Not appropriate:** Safe range is per dose not per 24 hours

C. What is the safe single dosage range?   _____

D. Is dosage ordered within a safe and therapeutic range? _____

E. How many mg should be given per dosage?   _____

F. What route should the ordered medication be given?   _____

G. How many mL of medication for IM use which will

then be diluted for IV use?   _____

H. Volume of fluid needed for maximum IV concentration? _____

> 25 DOSETTE® Vials
> Each contains **1 mL**
> **MORPHINE** CII
> SULFATE INJECTION, USP
> **10** mg/mL  **WARNING: May be habit forming.**
> FOR SC, IM OR SLOW IV USE
> NOT FOR EPIDURAL OR INTRATHECAL USE
> **PROTECT FROM LIGHT** — Store at 15°-30°C (59°-86°F). Avoid freezing.
> **USUAL DOSAGE:** See package insert.
>
> *NDC 0641-***0180-25**
> Each mL contains morphine sulfate 10 mg, monobasic sodium phosphate, monohydrate 10 mg, dibasic sodium phosphate, anhydrous 2.8 mg, sodium formaldehyde sulfoxylate 3 mg and phenol 2.5 mg in Water for Injection. pH 2.5-6.5; sulfuric acid added, if needed, for pH adjustment. Sealed under nitrogen. **NOTE:** Do not use if color is darker than pale yellow, if it is discolored in any other way or if it contains a precipitate. Caution: Federal law prohibits dispensing without prescription. Code: 0180-25 B-50180h
>
> **ELKINS-SINN, INC.** Cherry Hill, NJ 08003-4099
> *A subsidiary of A. H. Robins Company*

If your unit gives morphine sulfate frequently, **4 mg/mL** can be ordered. There is less chance of error when this concentration is used.

23. The physician orders Vancocin (vancomycin), 36 mg IV q8h. The child weighs 24 lbs, 10 oz. According to *The Harriet Lane Handbook,* the safe dosage for vancomycin is 10 - 15 mg/kg/24 hrs divided every 8 hrs. *The Pediatric Dosage Handbook* states that the safe IV concentration should not exceed 5 mg/mL and should be given over 60 minutes. The nurse adds 10 mL of diluent to the vial.

**Note:** *Vancomycin should not be given IM. Parenteral vancomycin is for IV administration only.*

A. What is the child's weight in kg?   _____

B. What is the safe 24 hour dosage range?   _____

C. What is the safe single dosage range?   _____

D. Is dosage ordered within a safe and therapeutic range?_____

E. How many mg should be given per dosage?   _____

F. What route should the ordered medication be given?   _____

G. How many mL of medication for IV use?   _____

H. Volume of fluid needed for maximum IV

concentration?   _____

I. What rate should the medication be delivered IV?   _____

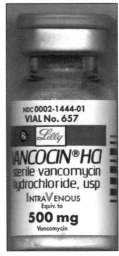

NDC 0002-1444-01
VIAL No. 657
℞ *Lilly*
VANCOCIN®HCl
sterile vancomycin
hydrochloride, usp
INTRAVENOUS
Equiv. to
**500 mg**
Vancomycin

Add 10 mL of diluent to yield 50mg/mL

24. The physician orders Unipen (nafcillin) 470 mg IV q6h. The child weighs 17.22 kg. According to *The Harriet Lane Handbook*, the safe dosage in infants and children is 100- 200 mg/kg/24 hrs divided every 6 hrs. *The Pediatric Dosage Handbook* states that intermittent infusion should be administered over 15 - 60 minutes at a final concentration not to exceed 40 mg/mL. The nurse adds 3.4 mL of diluent to the vial.

**Note:** *There is a high incidence of vein irritation with nafcillin. Due to this, nafcillin should be administered over 60 minutes and diluted as much as possible considering age, size vein, and physiologic status of the child. The physician may order sodium bicarbonate to be given with nafcillin to help decrease the incidence of vein irritation.*

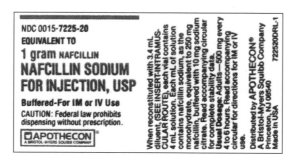

Add 3.4 mL of diluent to yield 1 g per 4 mL

A. What is the child's weight in kg? _____

B. What is the safe 24 hour dosage range? _____

C. What is the safe single dosage range? _____

D. Is dosage ordered within a safe and therapeutic range? _____

E. How many mg should be given per dosage? _____

F. What route should the ordered medication be given? _____

G. How many mL of medication for IM use which will then be diluted for IV use? _____

H. Volume of fluid needed for maximum IV concentration? _____

I. What rate should the medication be delivered IV? _____

25. The physician orders Cleocin (clindamycin) 210 mg IV q8h. The child weighs 46 lbs, 13 oz. According to *The Harriet Lane Handbook,* the safe dosage range is 20-30 mg/kg/24 hrs divided every 6 - 8 hrs. *The Pediatric Dosage Handbook* states that the safe intermittent IV concentration for clindamycin is 30 mg/mL and it should be given over 10 - 60 minutes.

A.  What is the child's weight in kg?                    _____

B.  What is the safe 24 hour dosage range?              _____

C.  What is the safe single dosage range?               _____

D.  Is dosage ordered within a safe and therapeutic range?    _____

E.  How many mg should be given per dosage?            _____

F.  What route should the ordered medication be given?      _____

G.  How many mL of medication for IM use which will then

    be diluted for IV use?                             _____

H.  Volume of fluid needed for maximum IV concentration?    _____

I.  What rate should the medication be delivered IV?       _____

Not for direct infusion.
For intramuscular or intravenous use.
See package insert for complete
product information.
Warning—If given intravenously, dilute before use.
Swab vial closure with an antiseptic solution.
Dispense aliquots from the vial via a suitable dispensing device into infusion fluids under a laminar
flow hood using aseptic technique. DISCARD VIAL
WITHIN 24 HOURS AFTER INITIAL ENTRY.
Store at controlled room temperature
15° to 30° C (59° to 86° F). Do not refrigerate.
Each mL contains: clindamycin phosphate equivalent to clindamycin 150 mg; also disodium edetate,
0.5 mg; benzyl alcohol 9.45 mg added as preservative. When necessary, pH was adjusted with
sodium hydroxide and/or hydrochloric acid.

813 718 403   DATE/TIME ENTERED ............

**Upjohn** NDC 0009-0728-05
6505-01-246-8718
60 mL Pharmacy Bulk Package

Cleocin Phosphate®
Sterile Solution

clindamycin phosphate
injection, USP

Equivalent to clindamycin

**150mg per mL**

Caution: Federal law prohibits
dispensing without prescription.

26. The physician orders Ancef (cefazolin), 56 mg IV every 8 hours. The infant weighs 5 lbs, 4 oz. According to *The Harriet Lane Handbook*, the safe dosage range for infants and children is 50-100 mg/kg/24 hours divided every 6-8 hours. *The Pediatric Dosage Handbook* states that the safe intermittent IV concentration for cefazolin is 20 mg/mL and it should be given over 10 - 60 minutes. The nurse adds 2.5 mL of diluent to the vial.

EXP.

**equivalent to**
**1 gram** cefazolin
*NDC 0007-3130-16*

**ANCEF**®
**STERILE CEFAZOLIN**
**SODIUM (LYOPHILIZED)**

**25 Vials for Intramuscular**
**or Intravenous Use**

LOT

NSN 6505-01-262-9508
**Before reconstitution protect from light and store at controlled room temperature (15° to 30°C; 59° to 86°F).**
**Usual Adult Dosage:** 250 mg to 1 gram every 6 to 8 hours. See accompanying prescribing information.
For I.M. administration add 2.5 mL of Sterile Water for Injection. SHAKE WELL. Withdraw entire contents. Provides an approximate volume of 3.0 mL (330 mg/mL). For I.V. administration see accompanying prescribing information.
Reconstituted *Ancef* is stable for 24 hours at room temperature or for 10 days if refrigerated (5°C or 41°F).
**SmithKline Beecham Pharmaceuticals**
Philadelphia, PA 19101          694115-N

K3130-16

Add 2.5 mL diluent
to yield 330 mg/mL

A. What is the infant's weight in kg? _____

B. What is the safe 24 hour dosage range? _____

C. What is the safe single dosage range? _____

D. Is dosage ordered within safe and therapeutic range? _____

E. How many mg should be given per dosage? _____

F. What route should the ordered medication be given? _____

G. How many mL of medication for IM use which will then

be diluted for IV use? _____

H. Volume of fluid needed for maximum IV concentration? _____

I. What rate should the medication be delivered IV? _____

27. The physician orders Wycillin (procaine penicillin) 450,000 Units IM q12h. The child weighs 40 lbs. According to *The Harriet Lane Handbook,* the safe dosage range is 25,000 - 50,000 Units/kg divided every 12 - 24 hours.

Note: *Procaine penicillin is for IM use only. It may not be given IV. Another form of penicillin would have to be used if penicillin were ordered IV.*

A. What is the child's weight in kg?  _____

B. What is the safe 24 hour dosage range?  _____

C. What is the safe single dosage range?  _____

D. Is dosage ordered within a safe and therapeutic range? _____

E. How many units should be given per dosage?  _____

F. What route should the ordered medication be given?  _____

G. How many mL of medication for IM use which will

then be diluted for IV use?  _____

H. Discard how many mL?  _____

**Wycillin**
(sterile penicillin G procaine suspension)

**1,200,000** units
**per TUBEX**

for deep **IM** injection only

Each TUBEX (2 mL size) contains
1,200,000 units penicillin G procaine in a
stabilized aqueous suspension with
sodium citrate buffer; and as w/v,
approximately 0.5% lecithin,
0.5% carboxymethylcellulose,
0.5% povidone, 0.1% methylparaben,
and 0.01% propylparaben.

Usual Dosage: See enclosed
information.

**Store in a refrigerator**
**Keep from freezing**

28. The physician orders Kefurox (cefuroxime) 700 mg IV q8h. The child weighs 34 lbs, 4 oz. According to *The Harriet Lane Handbook,* the safe dosage range for infants and children is 75 - 150 mg/kg/24 hrs divided every 8 hrs. *The Pediatric Dosage Handbook* states that safe intermittent IV concentration is 30 mg/mL and it should be given over 15 - 30 minutes. The nurse adds 3.6 mL of diluent to the vial.

A. What is the child's weight in kg? _____

B. What is the safe 24 hour dosage range? _____

C. What is the safe single dosage range? _____

D. Is dosage ordered within a safe and therapeutic range? _____

E. How many mg should be given per dosage? _____

F. What route should the ordered medication be given? _____

G. How many mL of medication for IM use which will then be diluted for IV use? _____

H. Volume of fluid needed for maximum IV concentration? _____

I. At what rate should the medication be delivered IV? _____

Add 3.6 mL of diluent
to yield 220 mg/mL

29. The physician orders ampicillin 200 mg IV q4h. The infant has meningitis and weighs 6 lbs, 10 oz. According to *The Harriet Lane Handbook,* the safe dosage range for infants with a severe infection is 200 - 400 mg/kg/24 hrs divided every 4 - 6 hrs. *The Pediatric Dosage Handbook* states that safe intermittent IV concentration is 30 mg/mL and it should be given over 15 - 30 minutes. The nurse adds 3.5 mL of diluent to the vial.

A. What is the infant's weight in kg? _____

B. What is the safe 24 hour dosage range? _____

C. What is the safe single dosage range? _____

D. Is dosage ordered within a safe and therapeutic range? _____

E. How many mg should be given per dosage? _____

F. What route should the ordered medication be given? _____

G. How many mL of medication for IM use which will then be diluted for IV use? _____

H. Volume of fluid needed for maximum IV concentration? _____

I. At what rate should the medication be delivered IV? _____

Add 3.5mL diluent
to yield 250 mg/mL

30. The physician orders tobramycin 65 mg IV q8h. The child weighs 60 lbs, 9 oz. According to *The Harriet Lane Handbook,* the safe dosage range for a child is 6 - 7.5 mg/kg/24 hrs divided every 8 hrs. *The Pediatric Dosage Handbook* states that safe intermittent IV concentration is 10 mg/mL and it should be given over 30 minutes.

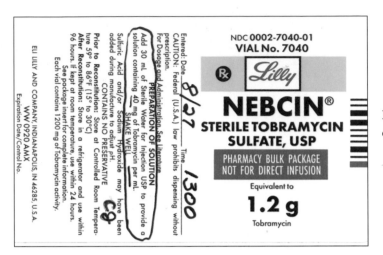

Reconstituted with 30mL of sterile water.

A. What is the child's weight in kg?  _____

B. What is the safe 24 hour dosage range?  _____

C. What is the safe single dosage range?  _____

D. Is dosage ordered within safe range?  _____

E. How many mg should be given per dosage?  _____

F. What route should the ordered medication be given?  _____

G. How many mL of medication for IM use which will then

   be diluted for IV use?  _____

H. Volume of fluid needed for maximum IV concentration?  _____

I. What rate should the medication be delivered IV?  _____

# Body Surface Area

The most reliable method of determining a child's dosage is to use estimated body surface area (BSA). The determination of body surface area requires the use of the West Nomogram Chart. Body surface area is estimated from height and weight and is expressed as meters square ($M^2$). This method is not used routinely for the calculation of medication dosages for children. It is used primarily for chemotherapeutic agents in the treatment of cancer in children and in other specialized areas. However, it can be used for many drugs. A reference text would identify the number of $mg/M^2$ as it identified the number of mg/kg for safe dosage ranges of certain medications.

## Body Surface Area based on West Nomogram Chart

The West Nomogram is a chart that uses height and weight to estimate body surface area.

Look at the chart. The height is on the left side of the chart and the weight is on the right side.

To determine body surface area:

1.  Place a ruler on the chart. Line up the ruler with the child's height on the left side of the chart and the weight on the right side of the chart.

2.  Read the BSA (body surface area) where the ruler intersects the BSA column. This gives the estimated surface area in $M^2$ (meters square).

Child's height is 32 inches (in)
Child's weight is 25 pounds (lbs)

What is the child's BSA?

Answer: 0.54 $M^2$

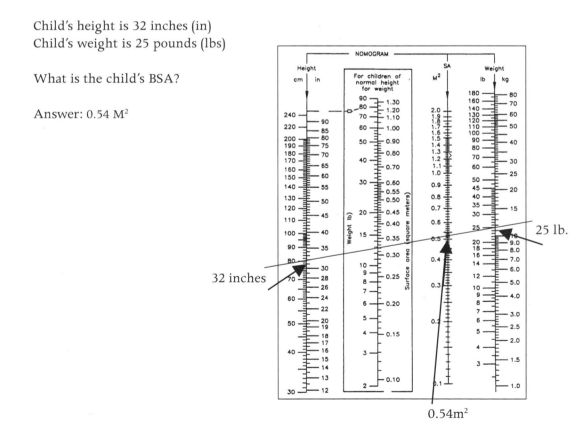

# West Nomogram Chart

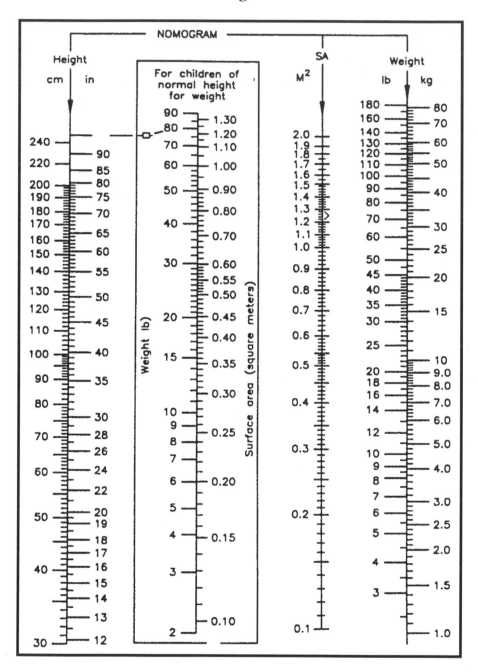

NOMOGRAM

**Height**

cm    in

**For children of normal height for weight**

Weight lb)

Surface area (square meters)

SA

M²

**Weight**

lb    kg

This chart is from *Nelson's Essentials of Pediatrics*, 1990 by Behrman and Kliegman, W.B. Saunders Company, Philadelphia. Reprinted by permission.

31.     Child's height:   18 in
        Child's weight:   6 lbs

        What is the child's BSA _____


32.     Child's height:   30 in
        Child's weight:   20 lbs

        What is the child's BSA _____


33.     Child's height:   22 in
        Child's weight:   10 lbs

        What is the child's BSA _____


34.     Child's height:   32 in
        Child's weight:   26 lbs

        What is the child's BSA _____


35.     Child's height:   170 cm
        Child's weight:   50 kg

        What is the child's BSA _____

**11.**
A   5.11 kg
B   1.53 mg/24 hrs
C   0.51 mg /dose
D   Yes
E   0.5 mg
F   Oral
G   1.3 mL
H   0.25 or 1/4 tsp
I   Yes

**12.**
A   6.59
B   19.77-39.54 mg/24hrs
C   6.59-13.18 mg /dose
D   Yes
E   9 mg
F   Oral
G   0.36 mL
H   Yes
I   Yes

**13.**
A   4.09 kg
B   81.8-163.6 mg/24 hrs
C   20.45-40.9 mg/dose
D   Slightly low, give as
    ordered, if not effective,
    notify physician
E   20 mg
F   Oral
G   1 mL
H   0.2 or 1/5 tsp
I   No, measurement in a
    syringe would be more
    appropriate

**14.**
A   3.30 kg
B   33-39.5 mcg/24 hrs
C   16.5-19.8 mcg/dose
D   Yes
E   18 mcg
F   oral
G   0.36 mL
H   Not appropriate

**15.**
A   12.61 kg
B   100.88-126.1 mg/kg/24 hrs
C   33.63-42.03 mg/dose
D   Yes
E   40 mg
F   Oral
G   1.6 mL
H   0.32 tsp
I   No, measurement in a syringe
    would be more appropriate

**16.**
A   9.32 kg
B   4.66-372.8 mg/24 hrs
C   2.33-186.4 mg/dose
D   Yes
E   150
F   Oral
G   30 mL
H   6 tsp or 2 T
    (3 teaspoons=1tablespoon)
I   Yes

**17.**
A   4.55 kg
B   182 mg/24 hrs
C   60.67 mg/dose
D   No, hold dose, notify physician.
E   Hold dose, DO NOT GIVE
F   Oral once dose is adjusted
G    7.2 mL would equal 180 mg
    but do not give
H   1.4 or 1 2/5 tsp would equal
    180 mg, but do not give
I   No, this is not a practical
    amount to measure in teaspoons

**18.**
A   15.91 kg
B   95.46-127.28 mg/24 hrs
C   47.73-63.64 mg/dose
D   No, dose is too low. Check
    with physician
E   45, but check with physician
F   Oral
G   11.3 mL, but check with
    physician
H   2.26 or 2 1/4 tsp, but check with
    physician
I   yes

**19.**
A   12.27
B   3.68 mg/24 hrs
C   1.23 mg/dose
D   Yes
E   1.2 mg
F   Oral
G   3 mL
H   0.6 or 3/5 tsp
I   No, measurement in a syringe
    would be more appropriate

**20.**
A   27.27
B   Not applicable -Safe range is per
    dose not per 24 hrs
C   272.7-409.05 mg/dose
D   No. Dose is low, give as ordered,
    if dose is not effective, notify
    physician
E   240 mg/dose
F    Oral
G   7.5 mL
H   1.5 tsp
I   yes

**21.**
A   10.34 kg
B   62.04-77.55 mg/24 hrs
C   20.68-25.85 mg/dose
D   Yes
E   25 mg
F   IV
G   0.63 mL
H   2.5 mL
I   5 mL/hr or gtts/min

**22.**
A   25 kg
B   Not appropriate, safe range is
    per dose
C   2.5-5 mg/dose
D   Yes
E   5 mg
F   IV
G   0.5 mL
H   1 mL

Answers: Chapter 7, *continued*

**23.**
A  11.19 kg
B  111.9-167.85 mg/24 hrs
C  37.06-55.95 mg/dose
D  No, dose is low, check vancomycin peak and trough levels. Do appropriate checks
E  36 mg
F  IV
G  0.72
H  7.2
I  7.2 mL/hr or gtts/min

**24.**
A  17.22 kg
B  1722-3444 mg/24 hrs
C  430.5-861 mg/dose
D  Yes
E  470 mg
F  IV
G  1.9 mL
H  11.8 mL (diluted as much as possible considering age, size of vein, & physiologic status).
I  11.8 mL/hr or gtts/min (should be given in maximum recommended time of 60 minutes)

**25.**
A  21.28 kg
B  425.6-638.4 mg/24 hrs
C  141.9-212.8 mg/dose
D  Yes
E.  210 mg
F  IV
G  1.4 mL
H  7 mL
I  7-42mL/hr or gtts/min

**26.**
A  2.39 kg
B  119.5-239 mg/24 hrs
C  39.83-79.67 mg/dose
D  Yes
E  56
F  IV
G  0.17 mL
H  2.8 mL
I  2.8-16.8 mL/hr or gtts/min

**27.**
A  18.18 kg
B  454,500-909,000 Units/24 hrs
C  227,250-454,500 Units/dose
D  Yes
E  450,000
F  IM
G  0.75 mL
H  1.25 mL

**28.**
A  15.57 kg
B  1167.75-2335.5 mg/24 hrs
C  389.25-778.5 mg/dose
D  Yes
E  700 mg
F  IV
G  3.2 mL
H  23.3 mL
I  46.6-93.2 mL/hr or gtts/min

**29.**
A  3.01 kg
B  602-1202 mg/24 hrs
C  100.33-200.67 mg/dose
D  Yes
E  200
F  IV
G  0.8 mL
H  6.67 mL
I  13.3-26.7 mL/hr or gtts/min

**30.**
A  27.53 kg
B  165.18-206.48 mg/24 hrs
C  55.06-68.83 mg/dose
D  Yes
E  65 mg
F  IV
G  1.6 mL
H  6.5 mL
I  13 mL/hr or gtts/min

31. $0.19 \text{ M}^2$

32. $0.45 \text{ M}^2$

33. $0.27 \text{ M}^2$

34. $0.53 \text{ M}^2$

35. $1.55 \text{ M}^2$

## References:

Green, M.G. (1993). *The Harriet Lane Handbook* (14th ed.). Chicago: Yearbook Medical.

*Physicians' Desk Reference*. (1993). Montvale, NJ: Medical Economics Date.

Taketomo, C.K., Hodding, J.H. & Kraus, D.M. (1993). *Pediatric Dosage Handbook* (2nd ed.). Chicago: Lexi-Comp, Inc.

# Notes

# 8

# Chapter Eight

# Intravenous Infusion Rates

# Intravenous Infusion Rates

## Introduction
This chapter will discuss some general concepts in administering fluids, blood and total parenteral nutrition (TPN). Sample problems will show how to calculate drops per minute and milliliters per hour. There will be practice problems to work.

## IV Therapy
Intravenous fluids are given for the following reasons.
1. **Fluid maintenance,** on a daily basis, can range from 1500-2500 mL per day in the adult patient. If the patient can not take that amount of fluid by mouth, then fluid maintenance can be achieved by intravenous therapy. An example of fluid maintenance is routinely ordering IV fluids preoperatively for all surgical patients

2. **Fluid replacement** is extra fluids given in addition to fluid maintenance to replace loss through diarrhea, nasogastric tubes, drains, burns and fever. Example of fluid replacement: An IV is ordered for a patient who has had several days of diarrhea and vomiting. Fluids are replaced along with specific electrolytes that are lost with diarrhea and vomiting.

3. **Glucose and electrolytes** are given to maintain fluid and electrolyte balance.

## Determination of IV fluids needed
Daily fluid maintenance requirement for an adult for both sensible and insensible loss is about 1500-2500 mL per day. The physician orders from 1500-2500 mL per day plus additional amounts for losses from drains, fever, and nasogastric tubes.

## IV orders
The physician individualizes the fluid for each patient by reviewing the intake and output record, the patient's weight, and serum electrolytes.

The physician's order must specify:
1. **The type of fluid**
   The type of fluid is Dextrose 5% in Water (D5W) alternate with Ringers Lactate (RL)
2. **The amount of IV fluid**
   The amount is for 1000 mL q10h or 2400 mL per day
3. **The rate of flow**
   The rate is 100 mL/h

> ### Physician's Order
>
> 3/5/__  D5W alternate with RL
>
> 1000 mL q10h
>
> Dr. Delvicario

## Common types of fluids
There are numerous types of intravenous fluids available. The ones described next are utilized most commonly.

**Note:** *The bags look similar at a glance. Read the label three times very carefully.*

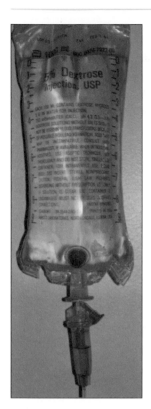

## 5% Dextrose and Water (D5W)

D5W is a hypotonic solution used to provide calories and water for hydration. Although the patient may be eating and taking fluids normally, venous access is readily available should a sudden change in the patient's condition occur. D5W is the fluid of choice for cardiac patients, who are on restricted sodium intake and need IV access for administration of medications.

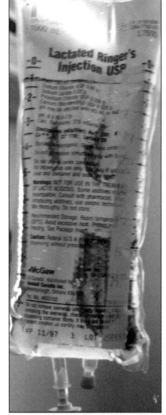

## Lactated Ringer's (LR) and 5% Dextrose and Lactated Ringer's (D5LR)

LR and D5LR are balanced solutions for hydration and maintenance of electrolyte balance. They are used most frequently for fluid maintenance during and immediately after surgery when the patient is not taking fluids by mouth.

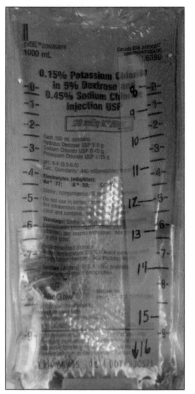

## 5% Dextrose and Normal Saline (D5 0.9NS) and 5% Dextrose and half Normal Saline (D5% 0.45NS)

D5 0.9NS and D5 0.45NS are also used post operatively for fluid maintenance when the replacement of some sodium is necessary.

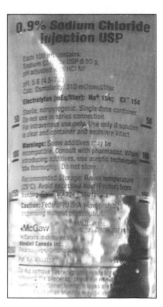

## Normal Saline (NS) and half normal saline (0.45NS)

NS and 0.45NS are saline solutions **without dextrose**. They are used frequently with diabetic patients who can not tolerate excessive amounts of glucose.

# IV Sites

## Peripheral

Peripheral IV sites are located in the superficial veins of the forearm, hand, and scalp of children. Peripheral leg veins should be avoided for IV therapy due to the risk of thrombophlebitis. A peripheral line can be used for short term IV fluid therapy and the administration of most antibiotics IV PB or IV push. Total parenteral nutrition with 10% Dextrose can be given in a peripheral vein.

## Central

Central IV sites are large veins like the **subclavian, external jugular, and femoral veins.** Central lines are inserted by the physician and are best for more irritating drugs, fast administration of blood or IV solutions in emergency situations, and for long term IV therapy. Total parenteral nutrition with 25% Dextrose must only be given through a central line. Many chemotherapeutic drugs may only be given though a central line.

## Central

A PICC Catheter (pheripherally inserted central catheter) is a long catheter insered in an antecubital vein with the tip positioned in the superior vena cava.

## Central

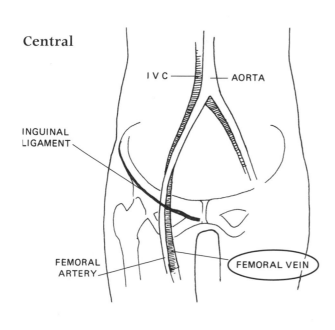

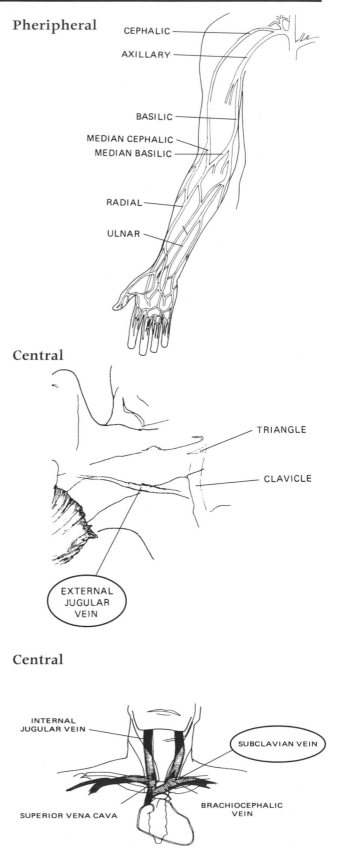

## IV Fluids

IV fluids are dispensed in plastic bags. Tubing is inserted into the bag. The tubing has a drip chamber. Pictured is a macrodrop tubing by IVAC with **20 drops per mL.** Other manufacturers of IV tubing may have different drop factors. The tubing has three injection ports for administration of drugs. There is also an access port in the bag of IV solution, where drugs may be added. Note the drip chamber where the drops from the IV bag can be counted. **The IV tubing is primed** by hanging the bag, squeezing the drip chamber until it is half full, opening the roller clamp and allowing the entire length of the tubing to fill with fluid without air bubbles and then closing the clamp.

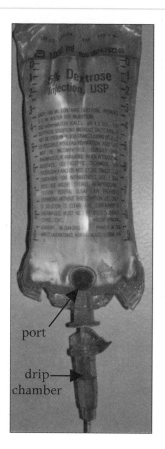

port

drip chamber

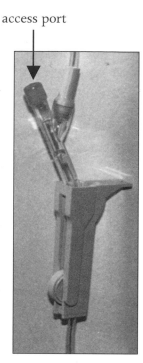

access port

roller clamp

Intravenous fluids can be administered two ways by either gravity or electronic pump. Gravity is used for short term IV therapy and when precise hourly intake is not absolutely critical. The electronic pump is used when precise maintenance of hourly intake is critical for titration of drugs, secondary IV PBs and for any central line infusion.

## Gravity flow

When gravity flow is used, the IV bag must hang higher than the patient's heart and the **higher the bag is hung the faster the IV will flow.** The **roller clamp** is adjusted to regulate the rate of flow, but the rate of flow will change when the patient changes position. IV fluids that employ gravity flow must be checked hourly or more often for readjustment of the infusion rate. The infusion rate can vary considerably with changes of position, from running too rapidly to not running at all. In summary, gravity IVs are "positional".

## Nurses responsibilities for IV flow rates for gravity are to:

- Determine the number of milliliters per hour that the patient should receive.

- Determine the drop factor of the IV tubing.

- Calculate the IV flow rate from mL per hour to drops per minute.

- Observe the drip chamber and regulate the rate of flow with the roller clamp until the number of drops per minute is correct.

**Note:** *This is determined by counting the number of drops for one minute.*

- Check the infusion rate hourly or more frequently if necessary.

## Drop Factor

The drop factor is the number of drops per mL and depends on the size of the opening in the drip chamber. IV tubings are not all alike. Tubing comes in various drop factors. The drop factor is indicated on the IV tubing package and varies from one company to another.

**Note:** *To determine the drop factor, read the IV tubing package.*

This tubing has a drip factor of 15 drops/mL

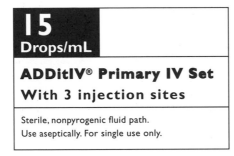

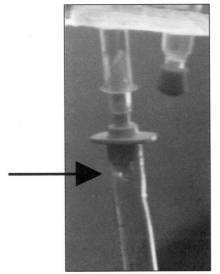

## Examples of 3 sizes of Macrodrop Tubings

Some IV drip chambers deliver 10 drops per mL, others 12 drops per mL and others 15 drops per mL. The amounts below are all considered macrodrops. Macrodrop means a large drop. Large amounts of IV fluids are administered in macrodrops. A general rule when administering more than 100 mL per hour is to select a macrodrop tubing.

### MACRODROPS

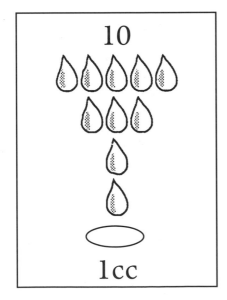

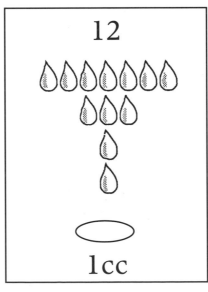

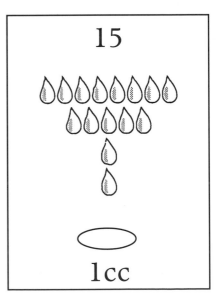

## Microdrip Tubing

Some IV drip chambers deliver 60 drops per mL. This amount is considered a microdrip. ML per hour and microdrops per minute with an Electronic Pump have the same rate of infusion. Most pump rates are set by mL per hour, but some are set by drops per minute.

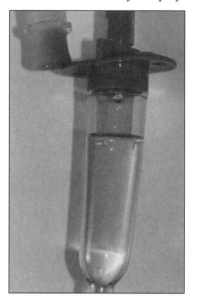

VENOSET® MICRODRIP®
## Piggyback Set, Nonvented, 78 Inch

**60** DROPS/mL

## Electronic Pumps

There are many brands of electric pumps available for IV fluid administration. The two ways the pumps work are **rate controllers** and **voluMetric controllers**. The IMed Gemini PC-1 can be set as either a rate controller or voluMetric pump by changing the mode button on the pump. It can be used for the administration of fluids, secondary piggybacks, drugs, and blood. The rate of the IV or drug can be set from 1-999 mL per hour. If the pump cannot maintain the set rate of infusion, it will alarm. With other brands, the nurse must select either a rate controller or a voluMetric controller. The company will designate different model numbers for each type of pump.

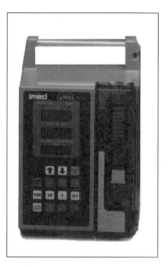

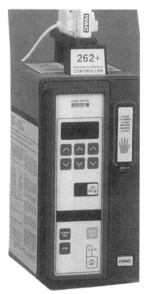

**Rate controller mode** of IV administration is the same principle as running the IV by gravity flow. The pump has a device that oscillates the tubing measuring the correct infusion rate.

**VoluMetric mode** of IV administration forces the fluid in against pressure and resistance. This type of pump is used for central venous lines and in rare cases when a drug needs to be infused into an artery.

The volumetric mode is IVAC's 570 model, which delivers in mL/h.

IVAC has a different pump for each mode of IV fluid administration. The rate controller mode is IVAC's 262 model, delivers in drops/minute.

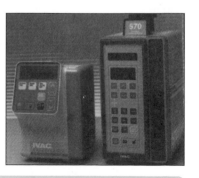

### Flow Guard

The newer pumps have flow guard or devices that protect against free flow when the door of the pump is opened. **This prevents the patient from receiving a large bolus of a drug or IV fluid when the door of the pump is opened. With the older models the IV runs wide open.** The roller clamp should be secured before opening the door of the pump, especially on the older models which do not have a flow guard.

**Note:** *As an extra precaution, whenever the door is opened or the tubing is changed, the roller clamp should be tightly secured in the off position. A large bolus of drugs can have very serious consequences for the patient. For example, a bolus of Nipride will cause the patient's blood pressure to bottom out to dangerously low levels. An R N who is familiar with the electronic pump should always accompany a patient who is being transported with a drug infusing on a pump.*

### Nurses Responsibility for IV administration using an electronic pump

- Be familiar with the proper operation of the pump.

- Only administer blood with an infusion pump that is designed to be used for blood. The older models of electronic pumps were not designed for administration of blood and can cause hemolysis of the red blood cells (RBC's).

- Plug in the pump so that it will remain charged for transportation of the patient on battery mode.

- Select the tubing that corresponds to the pump.

- Prime the IV tubing with IV fluid making sure to remove all air bubbles.

- Insert the tubing into the pump.

- Close the door.

- Determine the number of **mL per hour** to be administered and **set the correct rate.**

- Push start.

## Causes for the pump to alarm

1. Occlusion of the catheter
2. Open door to the pump
3. Air in the line
4. Low battery

## Causes of catheter occlusion

1. The catheter is no longer in the vein so the fluid is not freely infusing into the vein, but is into the subcutaneous tissue. This is evidenced by swelling and possible redness at the site. When this occurs, the IV must be stopped and the catheter discontinued. The IV can be resumed after a new IV catheter is inserted. Extravasation of some drugs into the tissue is a very serious problem and can cause sloughing and tissue necrosis. The patency of the IV should be checked at least every hour.

2. The patient has moved or bent the arm so the catheter is pinched or occluded. The arm may be repositioned and an arm board applied. Sometimes retaping the IV catheter helps.

3. A clot is in the catheter. When there is no blood return upon aspiration, there may be a clot at the cannula tip or along the vein wall. This can have serious consequences if the clot should break off with a life threatening embolism. The IV will need to be discontinued and restarted in another site.

4. Phlebitis is an inflammation of the vein and can cause partial occlusion of the flow. It is evidenced by a reddened streak along the vein, with tenderness, warmth, and edema at the venipuncture site. The venipuncture site should be inspected regularly. Discontinue the IV at the first signs of redness or tenderness and edema.

## Air in the line

1. Make sure the drip chamber is at least half full.

2. Aspirate the line with a syringe from the port distal to the air to remove the air.

3. Disconnect the line from the catheter using sterile technique and run the IV fluid through the tubing until all air is removed.

**Note:** *The drop factor is for gravity flow only. Each pump has IV tubing that is made specifically for the pump. Some pump tubing may be used for both gravity flow and electronic pump. Others may only be used in the pump. Regular IV tubing should be used for gravity flow, but if you switch to an electronic pump, the tubing will have to be changed to pump tubing.*

## Fluid Overload

Proper infusion rate of an IV helps to prevent fluid overload. Fluid overload occurs when too much fluid is delivered too fast. The symptoms of fluid overload are a rise in the central venous pressure (CVP), an increase in the blood pressure, shortness of breath, neck vein distension, and poor urine output. Maintaining a steady infusion rate helps to prevent fluid overload. However, fluid overload can occur regardless of the proper infusion rate with cardiac patients or patients with poor renal function. Should fluid overload occur, slow the IV to a KVO rate and notify the physician. The physician will probably order a diuretic such as Lasix and may change the infusion rate to a lesser amount per hour.

## Dehydration

When the infusion rate is too slow the patient will not receive the necessary fluid and electrolytes per day to maintain fluid and electrolyte balance and may become or remain dehydrated.

## Infection Control

Infection is prevented by careful attention to aseptic technique in care of the venipuncture site, IV solutions, and IV tubing. The fewer times a line is opened or manipulated, the lower the risk of infection. Catheter related sepsis is primarily a result of migration of organisms into the subcutaneous tissue of the catheter tract with resultant colonization of the catheter tip. The following are general guidelines for catheter care. Variations exist from one facility to another, so careful examination of the IV policy is necessary.

## General guidelines for catheter care

Change IV dressing everyday and assess site for signs of infection or phlebitis.

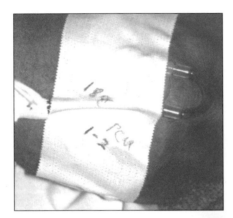

The transparent dressing allows easy observation of the catheter site.

The traditional gauze and tape dressing is most effective in areas that can be kept clean and dry. It is the least expensive dressing.

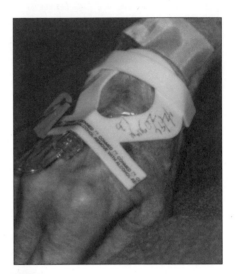

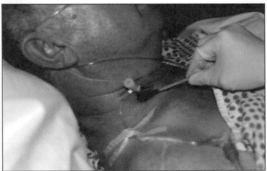

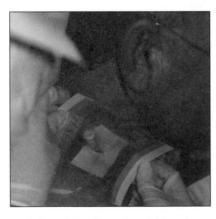

The OP-SITE dressing provides better visibility of the venipuncture site and is more occusive to contamination by tracheal secretions in the jugular site or by feces and urine in the femoral site. However, transparent dressing is more costly.

The IV tubing should be changed every three days and labeled with a sticker indicating the date and time the tubing is to be changed. Any IV solution should not hang for more than 24 hours.

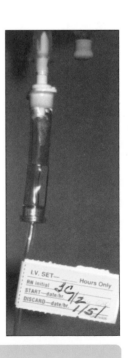

Peripheral IV sites should be changed every three days and central IV sites every five to seven days. The catheter tip of central lines is often sent to the lab for a culture and sensitivity to determine if colonization of the tip has occurred.

# Calculation of IV Drip Rate Using An Electronic Pump

■ The physician orders 1 L of D5W over 12 hours

**Formula mL/hour:**

$$\frac{\text{Total Volume to infuse (mL)}}{\text{Time (h)}} = \text{mL/h}$$

1 L = 1000 mL

$$\frac{1000 \text{ mL}}{12} = 83 \text{ mL/hour}$$

■ In summary, the electronic pump infusion rate must be set at 83 mL/hour.

# Calculation of IV Drip Rate Using Gravity Flow

■ The physician orders 1 liter of D5W over 12 hours (83 mL/h).

Drop factor 12 drops = 1 mL

**Formula: Flow rate drops/minute:**

$$\frac{\text{Volume in mL/h x drop factor}}{60 \text{ minutes/h}} = \text{Flow rate in drops per minute}$$

$$\frac{83 \text{ x } 12}{60} = \frac{996}{60} = 16.6 \text{ or } 17 \text{ drops per minute}$$

■ In summary, 17 drops per minute will deliver 83 mL per hour.

## IV Flow Rates for Piggyback Medication per Gravity

■ The patient is to receive Zincef 1 g in 50 mL D5W over 30 minutes.

Drop factor: 15 drops = 1 mL

**Formula:**

$$\frac{\text{Volume in mL x drop factor}}{\text{Time in minutes}} = \text{Flow rate in drops / minute}$$

$$\frac{50 \text{ mL x } 15 \text{ gtts}}{30 \text{ minutes}} = \frac{750}{30} = 25 \text{ gtts per minute}$$

■ In summary, 25 gtts per min will deliver 50 mL D5W over 30 minutes.

## IV Flow Rate of Piggyback Medication Using an Electronic Pump

■ The patient is to receive Zincef 1 g in 50 mL of D5W over 30 minutes.

**Note:** *The drug is ordered over 30 minutes rather than 1 hour. Electronic pumps infusion rates are set in mL per hour.*

**Formula:**

$$\frac{50 \text{ mL}}{30 \text{ min}} = \frac{\text{X mL}}{60 \text{ mins}}$$

$$30 \text{ X} = 3000$$

$$\text{X} = 100 \text{ mL/h}$$

$$1g \cdot \frac{50ml}{.5}$$

■ In summary, the electronic pump would be set at 100 mL per hour to infuse the 50 mL of Zincef in 30 minutes.

# Simple Method for Calculating IV Drip Rate With Microdrip Tubing

■ The number of drops per minute will equal the number of mL's per hour that the patient will receive. If the physician's order is to give 75 mL per hour with a microdrip, the IV would run at 75 drops per minute.

If the physician orders 60 mL per hour, the IV would run at 60 drops per minute.

If the physician's order is to run the IV at 20 mL per hour, the IV would run at 20 drops per minute.

20 mL / hour = 20 microdrops / minute
25 mL / hour = 25 microdrops / minute
30 mL / hour = 30 microdrops / minute
35 mL / hour = 35 microdrops / minute

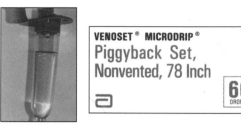

Drop Factor: 60 drops = 1 mL
Use the formula for IV calculation to illustrate that 75 mL / hour equals 75 microdrops / minute

$$\frac{\text{mL per hour x drop factor}}{\text{Number of minutes}} = \text{microdrops per min}$$

**Note:** *Microdrops / minute = mL / hour*

$$\frac{75 \times 60}{60} = 75 \text{ microdrops per minute}$$

■ **In summary, 75 mL per hour = 75 microdrops per minute**

# Infusion Time

■ 1000 mL of D5W is to infuse at 125 mL / h. How many hours will it take for this liter of fluid to be completed?

**Formula for Infusion Time**

$$\frac{\text{Total volume to infuse}}{\text{mL / h}} = \text{infusion time (h)}$$

$$\frac{1000 \text{ mL}}{125 \text{ mL/h}} = 8 \text{ hours}$$

■ **In summary, 1000 mL at 125 mL/hour will take 8 hours.**

# Monitoring Intravenous Fluid Levels When Not Using an Infusion Pump

### Marking the Bag With Tape

The nurse sets the infusion rate (IR) by using a watch and counting the drops for 15 seconds and then multiplying by 4. The rate is adjusted by moving the roller clamp up or down accordingly.

The IV illustrated is 1000 mL to run at 100 mL per hour. The drop factor for the IV tubing is 15 drops/mL. The IR rate is 25 drops per minute. The nurse counts the IV rate for 15 seconds and adjusts it to 6 drops x 4 = 24 drops per minute.

The flow rate of an IV should be monitored every hour because the rate can vary when a patient moves his arm or is repositioned.

A tape placed on the IV bag or bottle helps the nurse to monitor the progress of the IV hourly.

A piece of the tape is placed next to the calibrations on the bottle or bag. The time the bottle was hung was 0700 and the patient is to receive 100 mL per hour. The markings on the tape make it easier for the nurse to monitor the IR every hour. The nurse checks the bottle at 1100.
Is the bottle on time? _____

Answer: No. It should have 600 mL left at 11AM.

The nurse must recalculate the IV rate to have it finish at 5 pm.

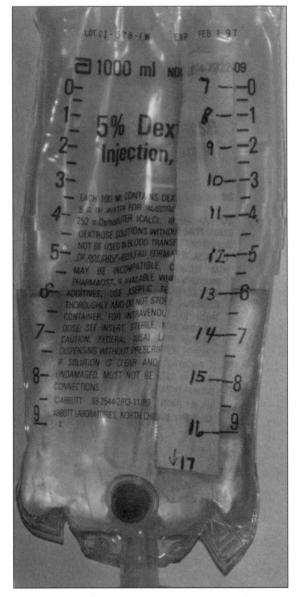

600mL infused - 400mL left

$$\frac{\text{Volume remaining}}{\text{Time remaining}} \quad \frac{400 \text{ mL}}{6 \text{ hours}} = 67 \text{ mL per hour}$$

$$\frac{67 \times 15}{60} = 17 \text{ drops per minute}$$

■ **In summary, slow the IV from 25 to 17 gtts/minute.**

## IV Fluids & Abbreviations

In abbreviations for fluids, D means dextrose, W means water, S means saline, NS means normal saline and the numbers indicate the percentage strengths. Become familiar with the abbreviations in the following chart.

### IV Fluids & Abbreviations

| | |
|---|---|
| D5W | 5% Dextrose and Water |
| D10W | 10% Dextrose and Water |
| D5NS | 5% Dextrose and 0.9% Normal Saline |
| D5 0.45NS | 5% Dextrose and Half Normal Saline |
| D5 0.2NS | 5% Dextrose and Quarter Normal Saline |
| RL | Ringer's Lactate |
| D5RL | 5% Dextrose and Ringer's Lactate |
| NS | 0.9% Normal Saline |
| 0.45NS | Half Normal Saline |
| 0.2NS | Quarter Normal Saline |
| KCl | Potassium Chloride |

*Practice Problems*

## Crystalloids

The following problems are for IV fluids, also called crystalloids. A crystalloid is a substance capable of crystallization, such as salt and sugar, which in a solution can diffuse through animal membranes. Patients who are receiving intravenous fluids must have both the intake and output monitored.

## Practice Problems IV Fluids

Calculate the infusion rate first for gravity flow and then for electronic infusion pump. Round off the answer to the nearest whole number.

1. The physician orders 1000 mL of D5W over 8 hours.
   Drop factor: 12 drops = 1 mL

   a. The IV is infused by gravity. Calculate the flow rate in drops/min.     _____

   b. The IV is infused by pump. Calculate the flow rate in mL/h     _____

2. The physician orders 1000 mL of D5W over 10 hours.
   Drop factor: 15 drops = 1 mL

   a. The IV is infused by gravity. Calculate the flow rate in drops/min.     _____

   b. The IV is infused by pump. Calculate the flow rate in mL/h     _____

3. The physician orders 1000 mL of D5 0.2NS with 20 KCl over 12 hours.
    Drop factor: 10 drops = 1 mL
    a. The IV is infused by gravity. Calculate the flow rate in drops/min.   $\underline{14 \text{ gtts}}$
    b. The IV is infused by pump. Calculate the flow rate in mL/h.   $\underline{83}$

$$\frac{1000 mL \times 10 d/mL}{12 \times 60 \ (720} = 13.8 \ (14) \quad \bigg/ \quad \frac{1000 mL}{12 hr}$$

4. The physician orders 500 mL NS over 8 hours.
    Drop factor: 15 drops = 1 mL
    a. The IV is infused by gravity. Calculate the flow rate in drops/min.   $\underline{16}$
    b. The IV is infused by pump. Calculate the flow rate in mL/h.   $\underline{63}$

$$\frac{500 mL \times 15 drop/mL}{8 \times 60 = 480 \ mm} \quad \frac{15.6 \ or}{16} \quad \frac{500 mL}{8 hr} \quad \frac{62.5}{63}$$

5. The physician orders 500 mL of RL over 5 hours.
    Drop factor: 10 drops = 1 mL
    a. The IV is infused by gravity. Calculate the flow rate in drops/min.   $\underline{17}$
    b. The IV is infused by pump. Calculate the flow rate in mL/h.   $\underline{100}$

$$\frac{500 mL \times 10 d/1 mL}{5 \times 60 \quad 300} \quad \frac{16.6}{17} \quad \frac{500 mL}{5 hr}$$

6. The physician orders 2500 mL of D5 0.45NS over 24 hours.
    Drop factor: 15 drops = 1 mL   drop factor
    a. The IV is infused by gravity. Calculate the flow rate in drops/min.   $\underline{\hphantom{xxxx}}$
    b. The IV is infused by pump. Calculate the flow rate in mL/h.   $\underline{\hphantom{xxxx}}$

$$\frac{2500 mL \times 15 drop/mL}{24 \times 60}$$

$$\frac{2500 mL}{24 \ hrs}$$

7. The patient is in hypovolemic shock. The physician orders 1000 mL of NS
    over 2 hours. Drop factor: 15 drops = 1 mL
    a. The IV is infused by gravity. Calculate the flow rate in drops/min.   $\underline{\hphantom{xxxx}}$
    b. The IV is infused by pump. Calculate the flow rate in mL/h.   $\underline{\hphantom{xxxx}}$

8. The physician orders 100 mL of NS over 20 min.
    Drop factor: 15 drops = 1 mL
    a. The IV is infused by gravity. Calculate the flow rate in drops/min.   $\underline{\hphantom{xxxx}}$
    b. The IV is infused by pump. Calculate the flow rate in mL/h.   $\underline{\hphantom{xxxx}}$

9. The patient's serum sodium is very low. The physician orders 250 mL of 3% hypertonic saline over 6 hours.
   The IV is infused by pump. Calculate the flow rate in mL/h. _____

**Note:** *Hypertonic solutions of sodium chloride should always be infused with a pump.*

$$\frac{25,000u \times 1800u}{500cc} \quad ?cc$$

$$25,000u \, ?cc = 1800u$$

$$500$$

10. The physician orders Vancocin 1 g in 150 mL of D5W over 1.5 hours.
    Drop factor: 60 drops = 1 mL
    a. The IV is infused by gravity. Calculate the flow rate in drops/min. _____
    b. The IV is infused by pump. Calculate the flow rate in mL/h. _____

11. The physician orders Ancef 1 g in 50 mL of D5W IV PB over 30 minutes.
    Drop factor: 15 drops = 1 mL
    a. The IV is infused by gravity. Calculate the flow rate in drops/min. _____
    b. The IV is infused by pump. Calculate the flow rate in mL/h. _____

12. The patient is to receive gentamicin 60 mg IV PB in 50 mL of D5W at 6 AM.
    The nurse set the flow rate on the infusion pump at 100 mL/h. What time will
    the IV PB be finished? _____

    top  Bottom

    $$\frac{50m/0.5}{100ml} \quad 6:30\ am$$

13. The physician orders 1000 mL of D5LR to run at 83 mL per hour.
    How many hours will 1 liter run? ____12hrs____

    $$\frac{1000mL}{83mC}$$

14. The patient's serum potassium is low, 2.8 mEq/L. The physician orders
    40 mEq of KCl in 250 mL of D5W to run over 4 hours.
    The IV is infused by pump. What is the rate of flow in mL/h? _____

**Note:** *Concentrated solutions of potassium should always be infused by pump not by gravity.*

$$\frac{250}{4}$$

15. The physician orders 1000 mL of D5 0.45NS with 20 mEq of KCl to run over 8 hours.
    Drop factor: 20 drops = 1 mL
    a. The IV is infused by gravity. Calculate the flow rate in drops/min. ____42____
    b. The IV is infused by pump. Calculate the flow rate in mL/h. ____125____

480

$$\frac{1000mL \times 20dr./1mL}{8 \times 60} \quad 480 \quad 41.6$$

$$42$$

$$\frac{1000}{8}$$

## Colloidal fluids

The following orders for IV fluids are called colloids. A colloid is a substance such as a protein or starch whose particles when dispersed in a solvent remain uniformly distributed and fail to form a true solution. The following IV fluids are used for hypovolemic shock and often are given rapidly, while careful monitoring of central venous pressure, blood pressure, and intake and output is required.

16. The physician orders Plasmonate 500 mL over 3 hours.
    Drop factor: 15 drops = 1 mL
    a. The IV is infused by gravity. Calculate the flow rate in drops/min.    _____
    b. The IV is infused by pump. Calculate the flow rate in mL/h    _____

17. The physician orders Plasmonate 250 mL over 2 hours.
    Drop factor: 12 drops = 1 mL
    a. The IV is infused by gravity. Calculate the flow rate in drops/min.    _____
    b. The IV is infused by pump. Calculate the flow rate in mL/h    _____

18. The physician orders Albumisol 25% in a 50 mL vial over 30 minutes.
    Drop factor: 10 drops = 1 mL
    a. The IV is infused by gravity. Calculate the flow rate in drops/min.    _____
    b. The IV is infused by pump. Calculate the flow rate in mL/h    _____

19. The physician orders 500 mL of Hespan over 4 hours.
    Drop factor: 12 drops = 1 mL
    a. The IV is infused by gravity. Calculate the flow rate in drops/min.    _____
    b. The IV is infused by pump. Calculate the flow rate in mL/h    _____

20. The physician orders Dextran 500 mL over 2 hours.
    Drop factor: 15 drops = 1 mL
    a. The IV is infused by gravity. Calculate the flow rate in drops/min.    _____
    b. The IV is infused by pump. Calculate the flow rate in mL/h    _____

21. You hung an IV of 1000 mL of D5W at 11 AM. The IV is to run 8 hours.
    What time should the IV be completed?    _____

22. A bag of 500 mL of D5 0.45NS is hung at 3 PM. The IV is to run at 100 mL/h.
    What time should this 500 mL bag be completed?  _____

23. The physician orders D5W at 50 mL/h.
    The 500 mL bag was hung at 12 noon. It is 3 PM.
    You check the bag at the beginning of your shift.
    You find 300 mLleft in the bag.
    Drop factor 15 drops = 1 mL

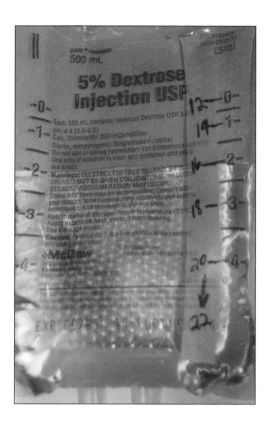

a. How much should have infused by 3 PM?  _____
b. How much has infused?  _____
c. Is the IV on time, ahead of time, behind time?
    Write the correct answer.  _____
d. What time should the IV be finished?  _____
e. How many mL are left in the bag?  _____
f. It is 3 PM. How many hours are left for
    the IV to finish on time?  _____
g. Calculate the infusion rate for the remaining
    amount of IV fluid in drops/min.  _____

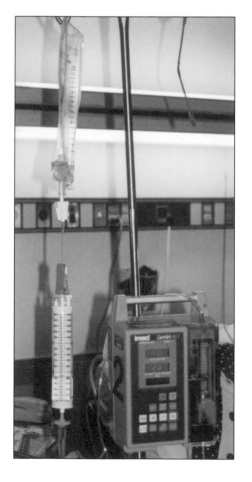

24. The physician orders 50 mL per hour of D5LR for a teenager with
    nephritis. At 12 noon you filled the soluset with 50 mL D5LR.
    At 1220 there is 45 mL left.
    Drop factor: 60 drops = 1 mL

    a. Is the IV on time, ahead of time,
        behind time?
        Write the correct answer.  _____

    b. Calculate the infusion rate for the remaining
        amount of IV fluid in drops/min.  _____

25. The physician orders 1000 mL D5 0.45NS + 20 mEq KCl at 125 mL per hour.
    Drop factor: 15 drops = 1 mL
    a. How many drops per minute would you give?  _____
    b. The liter was hung at 8 AM. It is now **1200 noon**. 600 mL was infused.
       Is the IV on time, ahead of time, or behind time?  Write the correct answer.  _____
    c. How much fluid should infuse by 1200?  _____
    d. What is the volume remaining?  _____
    e. How many hours are left for the IV to infuse on time?  _____
    f. Calculate the flow rate for the remaining amount of fluid in drops per minute.  _____

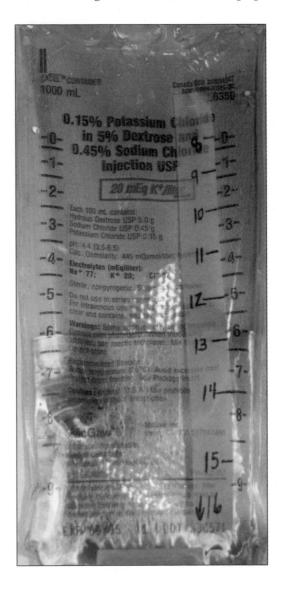

# Steps of Blood Component Administration

1. The physician writes an **order** for the transfusion of blood.

2. The order must be sent to the lab for **type and cross match**.

3. The nurse explains the purpose of the blood transfusion and has the patient sign the **consent** for the blood.

4. The lab draws blood for the type and cross match. The **blood specimen must be labeled immediately** with the patient's name, hospital identification number, the date and time the specimen was drawn. This needs to be signed by the person drawing the blood.

5. The nurse checks to see if the patient has an IV with a large bore catheter. A **number 18 gauge catheter** is needed for blood administration. If the patient has very small veins, a 20 gauge catheter can be used, but the blood will not run as freely.

6. Blood must be administered **with a filter** that removes debris and tiny clots found in the blood. A Y type blood tubing with a filter is used most often. The unit of blood is connected to one side of the Y and **a bag of normal saline** is connected to the other side. Only normal saline should be infused with blood. Prime the line with normal saline. Never use 5% Dextrose and Water with blood components. This can cause hemolysis of the cells.

7. Obtain the unit of blood from the blood bank after starting the IV and just before you are ready to administer the blood. **A unit of blood is only good for four hours after it is removed from the blood bank refrigerator.** All blood must be infused within four hours.

8. Know your hospitals protocol for blood administration. Strict adherence to procedure for blood administration prevents major hemolytic reactions that can occur when the wrong unit of blood is given to the patient. Check the order to be sure you have the right component. Then **two people must check the unit against the blood compatibility tag.** The ABO group of the patient's blood, and the RH type, must be the same as the unit of blood. Then check the expiration date on the unit of blood. Before hanging the blood, the **blood compatibility tag,** must be compared with the patient's arm band. The name and identification number should agree 100%. The blood cannot be administered if there is any discrepancy.

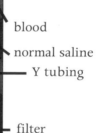

blood

normal saline

Y tubing

filter

9. After all pertinent information has been ascertained and the blood has been started, the unit must run slowly for the first 30 minutes. Most serious reactions will occur during this time. Hemolytic reactions are evidenced by flushing, fever, back pain, chest discomfort, headache, dyspnea, hypotension, hemoglobinuria, and oligura. Allergic reactions are characterized by chills, fever, and uticaria. If symptoms of transfusion reaction occur, stop the blood and keep the vein open with normal saline. Take the temperature and vital signs. Call the physician and blood bank. Follow the transfusion reaction protocol of the hospital.

26. The physician orders 1 unit (500 mL) of whole blood over three hours. A unit of blood is usually about a pint or 500 mL. The compatibility tag has been checked by 2 two nurses with proper identification of the patient. Base line vital signs and temperature have been obtained. For the first 30 minutes the blood is to run at 50 mL per hour.

    Drop factor: 10 drops = 1 mL

    The IV is infused by gravity. Calculate the flow rate in drops/min.    _____

27. The unit of blood has been running for 30 minutes. The vital signs and temperature are checked and found to be stable. You observe no signs of transfusion reaction such as fever, congestive heart failure, asthma, uticaria, or blood in the urine. The rate of flow is increased so 475 mL of blood is finished in about three hours.

    Drop factor: 10 drops = 1 mL

    The IV is infused by gravity. Calculate the flow rate in drops/min.    _____

28. The physician has ordered 1 unit of packed cells over four hours for Mr. Beach, who has a history of congestive heart failure. Packed cells is a unit of blood with about 250 mL of plasma removed. The patient is receiving the red blood cells without the extra fluid. This unit of packed cells contains approximately 270 mL.

    Drop factor: 10 drops = 1 mL

    The IV is infused by gravity. Calculate the flow rate in drops/min.    _____

29. The physician has ordered 1 unit of whole blood 550 mL to run over 2 hours. The unit has been running @ 50 mL per hour for 30 minutes. VS are stable with no evidence of transfusion reaction. A special blood pump is available and you use the pump to infuse the blood. 500 mL is left to run over 2 hours.

    The IV is infused by pump. Calculate the flow rate in mL/h.    _____

30. The physician has ordered 1 unit of packed cells to infuse over 2 hours. The unit is marked to contain 275 mL. The unit has been running at 50 mL per hour for 30 minutes. V.S. are stable with no evidence of transfusion reaction. The unit now contains 250 mL to run over 2 hours. You use the pump to infuse the blood.

    The IV is infused by pump. Calculate the flow rate in mL/h.    _____

# Total Parenteral Nutrition (TPN)

Regular IV fluids such as 5% Detrose and Water only provide fluids and carbohydrates. When oral intake is not possible or insufficient for an extended period of time, the patient will become malnourished. Total Parenteral Nutrition is the intravenous delivery of all essential nutrients such as protein, carbohydrates, fats, electrolytes, trace elements, and vitamins.

Total Parenteral Nutrition (TPN) is used:

1. When the gastrointestinal tract is not functioning and needs a rest such as with ulcerative colitis, and fistulas.

2. For critically ill patients who can not tolerate tube feedings.

3. For surgical patients, who are critically ill and can not tolerate tube feedings.

## Components of TPN

1. **Carbohydrates:** The final concentration of glucose is 25% or 250 g per liter of carbohydrates. Because it is a hypertonic solution it requires a central intravenous line, where it is infused into a large vein and dispersed rapidly into the vascular system.

2. **Protein:** Most TPN solutions contain about 40g of amino acid. The amount can vary to meet the individual needs of the patient.

3 **Fats:** The fats are given separately in the form of **10% lipid solutions.** A 500 mL bottle is hung piggyback to the TPN as the physician orders to meet the caloric needs of the patient.

4. **Vitamins:** Multivitamins (MVI) may be added to one liter bag daily.

5. **Trace elements** such as zinc, manganese, iodine, copper and chromium, are also added to the TPN.

## Administration of TPN

1. The patient must have a **central venous catheter for administration of TPN with 25% glucose.** Multilumen catheters are used frequently to provide a separate port for administration of other drugs. Medications should not be given with TPN due to the high probability of incompatibilities.

2. **The pharmacy should prepare the TPN** using meticulous sterile technique under a laminar flow hood. The high glucose concentration makes an excellent medium for the growth of bacteria. Infection and septicemia are the most common complications of TPN.

3. Before hanging TPN check the solution with the physician's order for TPN. Many hospitals have protocols for standard TPN solutions, but the physician may individualize the order for a particular patient.

4. A **filter, 0.22 micro,** must be used with TPN. It removes some microorganisms, vents air, and filters crystals out of the solution. The filter can not be used with lipids. If the lipids are infused, piggyback to the TPN and use a port below the filter for the TPN.

5. A **volumetric pump** must be used for administration of TPN.

6. **TPN must be started and stopped gradually.** Due to its high concentration of glucose it can cause hyperglycemia when it is started, and hypoglycemia if it is stopped suddenly.

7. With Total Nutrient Admixture (TNA) solutions the lipids, electrolytes, and trace elements, are added to the bag with the TPN solution for a 24 hour period. The TNA solution contains from 2000 to 3000 mL in a single bag. It simplifies the process and requires only one pump for its administration. The disadvantage of using TNA is if any changes in the composition of the TPN mixture need to be made, the entire day's supply needs to be discarded.

## Nursing assessment and monitoring

- Monitor blood sugar levels (fingerstick blood sugars) q6h when TPN is first started then once a day if there is no evidence of hyperglycemia. If the blood sugar is elevated, insulin may need to be added to the TPN.

Note: *If the physician had ordered the infusion rate to be cut in half to wean the patient from TPN and the finger stick blood sugar is normal, the TPN can be discontinued. If it is low, then the infusion rate should be cut in half again before discontinuing the TPN.*

- Monitor vital signs q6h and observe for fluid overload.

- Weigh the patient daily.

- Record intake and output carefully.

- Observe serum electrolytes, serum albumin, cholesterol, triglycerides, and liver enzymes. Report any abnormal results to the physician immediately.

- Change the tubing every 24 hours and carefully observe the venipuncture site for signs of infection or inflammation. Check temperature along with vital signs.

- Change dressing every 24 hours and carefully observe venipuncture site for signs of infection or inflammation. Check temperature along with vital signs.

### *Practice Problems*

31. The physician orders the standard TPN solution at your hospital. The protocol states to run 1 liter of TPN for the first 24 hours.
   The TPN is infused by volumetric pump. What is flow rate in mL/h?   _____

32. The physician orders the TPN to be increased to 2 liters per day.
   The TPN is infused by volumetric pump. What is the flow rate in mL/h?   _____

33. The patient has tolerated the TPN well with no evidence of hyperglycemia. The physician orders the patient to receive 3000 mL of TPN per day with multivitamins (MVI) added to 1 liter per day.
   The TPN is infused by volumetric pump. What is the flow rate in mL/h?   _____

34. The physician orders 500 mL of 10% Intralipids over 8 hours IV PB every other day. The lipid infusion has been inserted in a port distal to the filter.
   The lipids are infused by volumetric pump. What is the rate of flow in mL/h?   _____

35. The patient has been tolerating a full liquid diet by mouth. The physician orders the TPN to be weaned by cutting the infusion rate in half for one hour. The infusion rate has been 125 mL per hour.
   The TPN is infused by volumetric pump. What is half the flow rate in mL/h?   _____

36. Mrs. Jackson on home care is receiving 3000 mL of TNA per day. The TNA is infused by volumetric pump.
   Calculate the flow rate in mL per hour.   _____

# PCA Pump

### Patient Controlled Anlgesia (PCA pumps)

Patient controlled analgesia is a very useful tool for pain control for post operative and terminally ill patients. It allows a patient to administer the pain medication as needed by pushing a button.

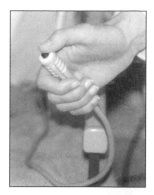

### PCA Syringe

The drug is contained in a large syringe (usually 60 mL) that is inserted into the PCA pump. The nurse must check the label for the concentration of the drug. The two drugs most commonly given per the PCA pump are morpine and meperidine (Demerol)

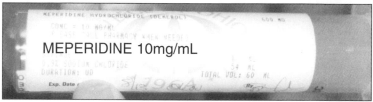

MEPERIDINE 10mg/mL

### Lock Out Interval

The pump is set with a "lock out" interval that is prescribed by the physician. If the "lock out" interval is every 15 minutes, the patients will receive a dose of the pain medication only every 15 minutes no matter how many times they push the button.

### PCA Dose

The PCA dose is the amount of pain medication given each time the patient pushes the button.

### Continuous Rate

The pumps can also be set to deliver a continuous rate of the drug per hour to prevent episodes of pain to occur when the patient is sleeping.

### Physician's Order

1.  The drug    **meperidine**
2.  The PCA dose        **10 mg/h**
3.  The lock out interval        **q 15 min**
4.  The continuous rate (optional)        **15 mg/h**

**Note:** *The physician may order only the PCA dose and not a continuous rate per hour.*

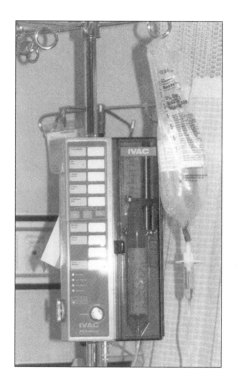

### Programming the PCA Pump

1.  Check the syringe for the concentration of the drug per mL......meperidine 10 mg/mL
2.  Set the PCA dose per hour......10 mg/h
3.  Set the lock out interval......q15min
4.  Set the continuous rate per hour...... 15 mg/h

**Note:** *Another nurse should double check the programming.*

### Nursing Assessment

| Level of Pain | Level of Consciousness (LOC) |
|---|---|
| 1.  None | 1.  Sleeping |
| 2.  Slight | 2.  Awake/alert |
| 3.  Tolerable | 3.  Awakens with stimulus |
| 4.  Moderate | 4.  Difficult to arouse |
| 5.  Severe | 5.  Disoriented |

**Note:** *Most hospitals provide pain management flow sheets for charting the above information.*

Answers: Chapter 8, 1-35

| | | | | | | | |
|---|---|---|---|---|---|---|---|
| 1. | a. | 25 | 14. | 63 | 24. | a. | behind |
| | b. | 125 | 15. | a. 42 | | b. | 68 |
| 2. | a. | 25 | | b. 125 | 25. | a. | 31 |
| | b. | 100 | 16 | a. 42 | | b. | ahead |
| 3. | a. | 14 | | b. 167 | | c. | 500 mL |
| | b. | 83 | 17. | a. 25 | | d. | 400 |
| 4. | a. | 16 | | b. 125 | | e. | 4 |
| | b. | 63 | 18. | a. 17 | | f. | 25 |
| 5. | a. | 17 | | b. 100 | 26. | 8 | |
| | b. | 100 | 19. | a. 25 | 27. | 26 | |
| 6. | a. | 26 | | b. 125 | 28. | 11 | |
| | b. | 104 | 20. | a. 63 | 29. | 250 | |
| 7. | a. | 125 | | b. 250 | 30. | 125 | |
| | b. | 500 | 21. | 7 PM or 1900 | 31. | 42mL/h | |
| 8. | a. | 75 | 22. | 8 PM or 2000 | 32. | 83mL/h | |
| | b. | 300 | 23. | a. 150 | 33. | 125mL/h | |
| 9. | 42 | | | b. 200 | 34. | 63mL/h | |
| 10. | a. | 100 | | c. ahead of time | 35. | 63mL/h | |
| | b. | 100 | | d. 10 PM or 2200 | 36. | 125 mL/h | |
| 11. | a. | 25 | | e. 300 | | | |
| | b. | 100 | | f. 7 hours | | | |
| 12. | 6:30 AM or 0630 | | | g. 11 | | | |
| 13. | 12 hours | | | | | | |

**References**

Folkes, Mary E. "Transfusion Therapy in Critical Care Nursing". Critical Care Quarterly 1990, 13 (2) p. 15-28.

Freedman, Sara E. "Tunneled Catheters - Technologic Advances and Nursing Care Issues". Nursing Clinics of North America. Vol. 28, Number 4, December 1993 p. 851-857.

Orr, Marsha Evans. "Issues in the Management of Percutaneous Central Venous Catheters". Vol. 28, Number 4, December 1993 p. 911-917.

Viall, Carolyn. "TPN Part One". Nursing 95. April p. 35-41

**9**

Chapter Nine

# Heparin

# Heparin

## Introduction

Chapter 9, Heparin, gives general information about why and how heparin is used, how to calculate the infusion flow rates, and concludes with practice problems.

Heparin is discussed separately in this book because its correct calculation is of primary importance. A precise therapeutic level of heparin is needed for the safety of the patient. The right amount of heparin prevents clot formation. Too much can cause bleeding.

## Heparin

Heparin is a potent anticoagulant that prevents clot formation and blood coagulation. Although it prevents the formation of a clot, it does not dissolve an existing clot. Heparin inactivates activated Factor X and inhibits the conversion of prothrombin to thrombin.

It also, in larger doses, inactivates thrombin and prevents the conversion of fibrinogen to fibrin. Heparin is used in the following clinical situations:
- thrombophlebitis
- post operative prosthetic valve replacement
- post operative angioplasty patients
- pulmonary emboli
- deep vein thrombosis
- atrial fibrillation with embolization

## Activated Partial Thromboplastin Time (APTT) and Heparin

The therapeutic range of heparin is determined by monitoring the patient's APTT. Before heparin therapy is started, and APTT should be drawn as the patient's baseline. The normal baseline APTT can vary in hospital labs from 16-35 seconds. (Usually for 10 second intervals such as 16 - 25 or 24 - 34)  Check with your facility for the baseline APTT.
The therapeutic range is 1.5 to 2.5 times the baseline APTT.

## Abbreviation
**Note:** *There has been evidence of errors when abbreviating the word unit. It is recommended that the word unit be written rather than abbreviated with the letter "u".*

## Administration of Heparin

Heparin is not given orally due to the fact that it is not absorbed well from the gastrointestinal tract. Heparin may be given the following ways.

1. By continuous intravenous infusion with an electronic infusion pump. This is the most common way heparin is administered because it provides a more constant degree of anticoagulation and less chance of bleeding. A heparin infusion is ordered in units per hour. For instance, the physician may order a heparin drip at 800 units per hour adjusted according to the lab results of the APTT.

2. Heparin may also be given as an intermittent intravenous infusion, however, bleeding complications occasionally occur with this method.

3. Intravenous heparin must be given in a separate line because it is inactivated by many other drugs.

4. Heparin, especially low dose prophylactic heparin, may be given subcutaneously.

**Note:** *Heparin may never be given intramuscularly due to the risk of hematoma.*

**Note:** *Some Heparin injections must be double checked with a second nurse and co-signed on the MAR.*

## Nursing Responsibilities
- Know how many units per hour are ordered.
- Know the results of the last APTT drawn and when the next one is to be drawn.
- Always recalculate the infusion rate to be sure it is accurate. Never assume that it has been calculated correctly. Examine the bag of heparin carefully to determine the number of units per mL.
- Notify the physician of the latest APTT results.
- Recalculate the infusion rate with any change in order based on the latest APTT.
- If the heparin infusion is stopped because the IV must be restarted, notify the physician, he may order a bolus of heparin IV in addition to resuming the heparin drip.
- Observe the patient for signs of bleeding, excessive bruising, hematuria and tarry stools.

## Premixed heparin

Heparin is now available in bags pre-mixed by the pharmaceutical company. Less chance of error occurs when the hospital uses a consistent concentration of the drug. A concentration of 25,000 units of heparin in a 250 mL bag is 100 units per mL. See the formula in the sample problem. However, always check the concentration of heparin on the bag. Heparin comes pre-mixed in more than one concentration.

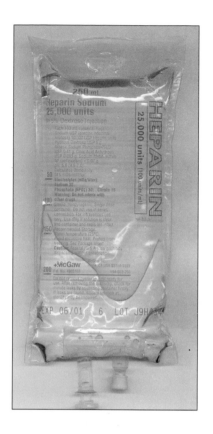

Abbott Laboratories carries heparin premixed in the following concentrations. Your hospital may only carry one or two of the concentrations available. This is why you must carefully read the bag for the concentration in that particular bag. Never assume that premixed heparin is 100 units/mL.

> ### Abbott Laboratories Premixed Heparin
>
> Heparin 25,000 units in 500 mL 0.45 NS-50 u/mL
>
> Heparin 25,000 units in 250 mL 0.45 NS-100 u/mL
>
> Heparin 12,500 units in 250 mL 0.45 NS-50 u/mL
>
> Heparin 20,000 units in 500 mL D5W - 40 u/mL
>
> Heparin 25,000 units in 500 mL D5W - 50 u/mL
>
> Heparin 10,000 units in 100 mL D5W - 100 u/mL
>
> Heparin 25,000 units in 250 mL D5W - 100 u/mL

Many cardiac patients are on fluid restrictions, and as a result the heparin may have to be mixed in a more concentrated solution to prevent fluid overload. However, there is more consistency in APTT results, with less concentrated heparin solutions. Greater consistency in APTT results occur when the same lot of heparin is used, and the coagulation instrument is calibrated to a single lot of heparin.

**Note:** *Enoxaparin (Lovenox) is the first low molecular weight heparin derivative marketed in the United States. Presently it may only be used for prevention of deep vein thrombosis after hip replacement surgery. It may eventually be approved for other uses. It is given subcutaneously and does not require the close monitoring of the APTT that heparin requires.*

# Ratio Proportion Method for Continuous Intravenous Infusion of a Drug Ordered per Hour

■ The physician orders heparin 800 units per hour.

Available from the pharmacy is a premixed bag of heparin 25,000 units in 250 mL

The IV is infused by pump. Calculate the flow rate in mL / h.  _____

Ratio Proportion Method

1,  Arrange the ratio proportion

$$\frac{25,000 \text{ units}}{250 \text{ mL}} = \frac{800 \text{ units}}{X \text{ mL}}$$

2.  Cross multiply the ratio proportion

25,000 X = 800 x 250

3.  Divide

$$X = \frac{200,000}{25,000}$$

X = 8 mL / h

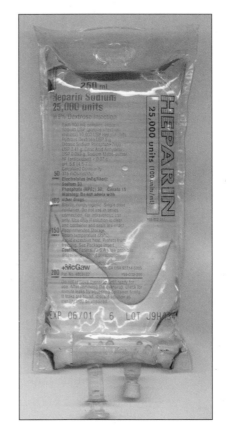

■ In summary, to give 800 units of heparin per hour, 8 mL per hour must be given.

# Formula Method for Continuous Intravenous Infusion of a Drug Ordered per Hour

■ **The doctor orders heparin 800 units per hour.**

Available from the pharmacy is a pre-mixed bag of heparin 25,000 units in 250 mL

The IV is infused by pump. Calculate the flow rate in mL / h _____

### Amount of the drug per mL

**Formula:**

$$\frac{\text{Known amount of drug (D)}}{\text{Total volume of diluent (V)}} = \text{Amount of drug / mL}$$

$$\frac{25,000 \text{ units}}{250 \text{ mL}} = 100 \text{ units per mL}$$

$$1 \text{ mL} = 100 \text{ units}$$

### Infusion Rate mL / hour

**Formula:**

$$\frac{\text{Dose / h desired}}{\text{Concentration / mL}} = \text{Infusion Rate (IR) mL/h}$$

$$\frac{800 \text{ units}}{100 \text{ units / mL}} = 8 \text{ mL / h}$$

■ **In summary, the infusion rate of 8 mL/h will deliver 800 units of heparin per hour.**

1.  Mrs. Lopez is admitted to the hospital one week after having a baby. She complains of pain in her left leg. The diagnosis is acute thrombophlebitis. Her physician places her on a heparin drip at 1000 units per hour initially.

    The bag is 250 mL of D5W. Read the label for the concentration of heparin.

    a.  What is the concentration of heparin in the bag?

    _____

    b.  What is the concentration of heparin per mL?

    _____

    c.  To give 1000 units of heparin per hour, the pump infusion rate is mL/h?

    _____

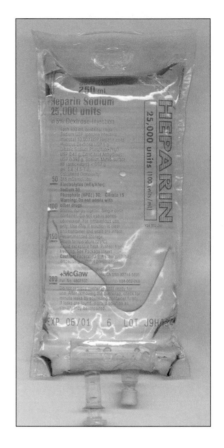

2.  An APTT is ordered to be drawn q4h for 24 hours. You have just received a lab report that indicates Mrs. Lopez's APTT is 56 seconds. The physician is notified of the results and the heparin drip is increased to 1300 units/hour. The concentration of heparin is the same. 25,000 units in 250 mL.

    To give 1300 units of heparin per hour, the pump infusion rate is mL/h?    _____

3.  In 4 hours another APTT is drawn from Mrs. Lopez. The result of the APTT is 100 seconds. The physician is called and orders the heparin stopped for two hours and then resumed at a drip rate of 900 units per hour.

    To give 900 units of heparin per hour, the pump infusion rate is mL/h?    _____

4. Mr. Jones is on a heparin drip for pulmonary emboli. The physician orders the heparin drip at 600 units per hour. The concentration is the standard pre-mixed heparin of 25,000 units per 250 mL of D5W. You have just started your shift and are making rounds. The pump infusion rate is set at 6 mL/h.

   a. What is the concentration of heparin per mL?  _____

   b. Is the heparin infusion rate correct?          Yes _____      No _____

5. Mr. Jones has an APTT ordered for 6 AM. The APTT result is 38. The physician orders an increase in the heparin drip to 1100 units per hour. The concentration of heparin remains 25,000 units in 250 mL of D5W.

   To give 1100 units of heparin per hour, the pump infusion rate is mL/h?  _____

6. Mr. Smith has a history of congestive heart failure and has currently been admitted for a pulmonary emboli. The physician orders a heparin drip at 600 units per hour.

   Read the label.

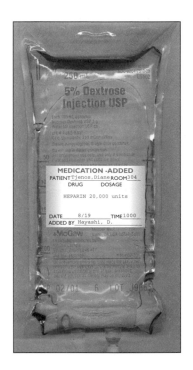

   a. What is the concentration of heparin in the bag?       _____
   b. What is the concentration of heparin per mL?           _____
   c. To give 600 units of heparin per hour, the pump infusion rate is mL/h?  _____

**Note:** *Patients who will need long term anticoagulant therapy will eventually be switched to Coumadin, an oral anticoagulant. Coumadin therapeutic levels are determined by the prothrombin time (PT). The heparin therapy is continued for several days after the Coumadin is initiated to ensure continuous anticoagulation therapy.*

7. Mr. Busen is scheduled for hip surgery and the physician orders heparin 5,000 units SQ 2 hours preoperatively for prophylaxis against postoperative deep vein thrombosis.
Read the label

Give? _____mL

**Upjohn NDC 0009-0317-01**
1 mL
**Heparin Sodium Injection, USP**
Sterile Solution
**10,000 Units per mL**
from beef lung

8. Mrs. Guyton has been admitted with the diagnosis of acute pulmonary emboli. The physician orders a bolus of heparin 10,000 units now, prior to starting a heparin drip.
Read the label

Give? _____mL

**Upjohn NDC 0009-0291-01**
10 mL
**Heparin Sodium Injection, USP**
Sterile Solution
from beef lung
**5,000 Units per mL**
For subcutaneous or intravenous use

9. The physician orders heparin 4,000 units SQ q8h for his bedridden patient.
Read the label.

Give? _____mL

**Upjohn NDC 0009-0317-01**
1 mL
**Heparin Sodium Injection, USP**
Sterile Solution
**10,000 Units per mL**
from beef lung

10. You need to flush a central venous line with heparin. Which of the two labels shown is appropriate for a heparin flush?

a. _____ or b. _____

a.
**Upjohn NDC 0009-0268-01**
10 mL
**Heparin Sodium Injection, USP**
Sterile Solution
from beef lung
**1,000 Units per mL**
For subcutaneous or intravenous use

b.
25 DOSETTE® Vials NDC 0641-**0387-25** 6505-01-194-7282
Each contains **2 mL**
**HEP-LOCK®**
HEPARIN LOCK FLUSH SOLUTION, USP
**100 units/mL**
FOR IV FLUSH ONLY
NOT FOR ANTICOAGULANT THERAPY
Each mL contains heparin sodium 100 USP units, sodium chloride 9 mg and benzyl alcohol 0.01 mL in Water for Injection. pH 5.0-7.5; sodium hydroxide and/or hydrochloric acid added, if needed, for pH adjustment. Sealed under nitrogen. Intended for maintenance of patency of intravenous injection devices only. Will alter results of blood coagulation tests. Nonpyrogenic. FROM PORCINE INTESTINES. Store at 15°-30°C (59°-86°F).
USUAL DOSAGE: See package insert.
Caution: Federal law prohibits dispensing without prescription. Code: 0387-25 B-50387h
esi ELKINS-SINN, INC. Cherry Hill, NJ 08003-4099
A subsidiary of A. H. Robins Company

Answers: Chapter 9, 1-10
1. a. 25,000 / 250 mL    4. a. 100 units    7. 0.5 mL
   b. 100                   b. Yes            8. 2 mL
   c. 10 mL / h          5. 11 mL / h        9. 0.4 mL
2. 13 mL / h            6. a. 20,000        10. b
3. 9 mL / h               b. 80 units / mL
                          c. 8mL

**10**

Chapter Ten

# Insulin Drug Calculation

# Insulin

### Introduction
This chapter includes: a description of insulin, the sources of insulin, categories of insulin, nursing responsibilities, insulin syringes, sample problem and practice problems.Insulin is discussed separately in this workbook because it is ordered in units, uses a special syringe to measure the dosage, and requires careful monitoring of the blood sugar in response to the insulin.

### What is Insulin?
Insulin is a natural hormone produced by the pancreas to maintain the body's blood sugar within the normal range of 80-120 mg/dL or 70-110 mg/dL, depending on the laboratory's normal range. It was first isolated in 1922 for the treatment of diabetic patients. Diabetes occurs when the pancreas does not make enough insulin to meet the body's needs. Insulin promotes the entry of glucose into all cells. Without adequate insulin, the serum glucose level remains abnormally high. This is called hyperglycemia. Hyperglycemia is controlled by adjusting the insulin dosage to maintain a normal serum blood sugar. If the patient receives too much insulin, hypoglycemia or a low blood sugar can occur.

### Sources of Insulin
In the past the main source of insulin came from animals. Human insulin, however, has replaced animal sources. Pork insulin is used infrequently. See below.

### Human Insulin
Human insulin is synthesized using a laboratory strain of Escherichia coli bacteria that has been genetically altered by addition of a gene for human insulin production. Recombinant, for the production of human insulin, DNA technology is replacing insulin isolated from pork and beef. Humulin is Eli Lilly's trade name for human insulin.

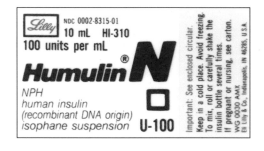

### Pork Source of Insulin
Pork insulin comes from a single source and is useful for patients who may have an insulin allergy or insulin resistance. An example of a single source pork insulin is Iletin II from Eli Lilly.
**Note:** *Beef insulin has been discontinued.*

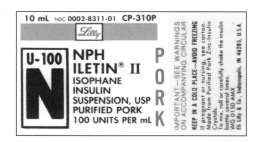

### Categories of Insulin
Insulin can be divided into four categories of action: short, rapid, intermediate, and long acting.

## Short acting insulin

Regular insulin is a short acting insulin. Its onset of action is ½ hour to 1 hour. Its maximum effect occurs in 2-4 hours and its duration of action is 6-8 hours. The regular insulin label has a large **R**, to distinguish it from other types of insulin. Regular insulin is a **clear colorless** liquid and is the only **insulin that may be given intravenously**. Regular insulin is also used when a diabetic patient is not eating or the blood sugar is out of control with conditions such as infection, and influenza.

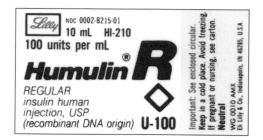

## Rapid acting insulin

Humalog insulin is the shortest acting insulin. This insulin starts to work very rapidly (within 15 minutes of administration) and its duration of action is less than 5 hours. When used as meal-time insulin, Humalog insulin must be given 15 minutes before a meal where as Regular insulin is given 30-60 minutes before a meal. Humalog insulin is intended for subcutaneous administration and its more rapid action is related to its quicker absorption from the subcutaneous tissue.

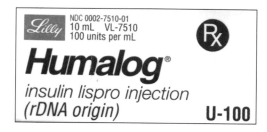

## Intermediate acting insulin

NPH insulin is intermediate in its length of action. Its onset of action is 1/2 hour, its maximum effect is 2-12 hours, and its length of action is 24 hours. The NPH insulin label has a large **N**, to distinguish it from other types of insulin. NPH looks uniformly cloudy when mixed. NPH insulin is often mixed with regular insulin and given twice a day before breakfast and dinner. This method of insulin administration more closely mimics the action of the pancreas, resulting in more consistent blood sugars.

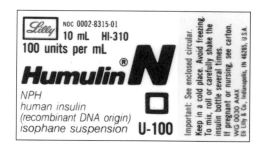

Humulin 70/30 is Eli Lilly's commercially prepared human insulin that is a mixture of **70% NPH** insulin and **30% Regular insulin**. The patient does not have to mix the insulin and it is administered twice a day before breakfast and dinner. The human insulin label has a large **70/30** to distinguish it from other types of insulin. It is an intermediate acting insulin and a short acting insulin.

## Intermediate acting insulin *cont.*

**Lente insulin** is another intermediate acting insulin. It also comes from beef/pork, pork, and human sources. The Lente insulin label has a large **L**, to distinguish it from other types of insulin. Its onset of action is 2 - 4 hours, peak action 6 - 12 hour, and duration of action 18 - 26 hours.

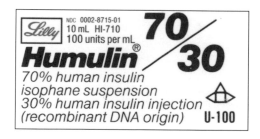

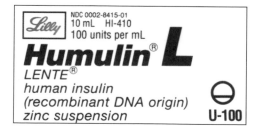

## Long Acting Insulin

**Ultralente** is a mixture of insulin that provides long action. The onset of action is not until 4 - 6 hours. The maximum effect is 8 - 20 hours and the duration of action is 24 - 28 hours. The Ultralente insulin label has a large U to distinguish it from other types of insulin.

## Lantus Insulin

Lantus insulin (insulin glargine) is the latest insulin on the market. The major difference of Lantus is that, once injected subcutaneously, it is absorbed slowly into the bloodstream with little variability and *no peak activity*. The duration of action is 24 hours, is administered at bedtime, and it may not be mixed with any other insulin.

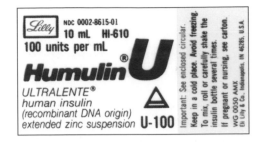

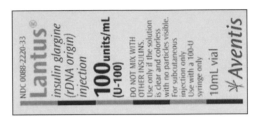

## Insulin Units

The potency of insulin is expressed in USP units per mL. The potency of insulin is standardized according to its ability to lower the blood glucose concentration of normal fasting rabbits as compared to the USP Reference Standard. Insulin is supplied in concentrations of **100 units per mL**. It is also supplied by Eli Lilly with 500 units per mL. This 500 units per mL concentration is only used for patients who require very large doses of insulin. In 1980 the production of U- 40 and U- 80 concentrations was discontinued.

> **Note:** *An insulin syringe can only be used for measuring insulin. Units are not interchangeable. A unit of insulin is not the same as a unit of heparin or penicillin. Do not use a Tuberculin syringe to measure insulin. Insulin syringes are designed with less dead space in the hub of the syringe.*

## Nursing Responsibilities

1. Determine the animal source of insulin the patient has been using.
2. Read the insulin label carefully to be sure that it is the same source of insulin that the patient has been taking. The physician may decide to change the source of the patient's insulin because of allergies or insulin resistance. When mixing insulin, be sure to use the same source of insulin for both regular and intermediate. When a patient is switched to a different insulin, they must be monitored carefully until the proper dosage is obtained to maintain the blood sugar within normal limits.
3. Determine that the insulin is the correct type of action such as short, intermediate or long acting.
4. Use U-100 insulin with an U-100 syringe. **Only use insulin syringes to measure insulin.**
5. Do finger stick blood sugars before administering the insulin or as ordered by the physician. A common order is finger stick blood sugars before meals and at bedtime. If the patient is not eating they may be ordered q6h.
6. Draw up the correct number of units of insulin being careful to get rid of any air bubbles.
7. Give the insulin at the scheduled time. Do not give intermediate or long acting insulin if the patient will not be eating at the regular times. Example: If the patient is NPO (nothing by mouth) before X-Ray or surgery, their usual morning insulin will not be given and the physician will need to be contacted for an adjustment of the dosage after the procedure is completed. Patients are often switched to sliding scale insulin until they resume their regular meal schedule.
8. Chart the blood sugar results and insulin administration on the diabetic record as well as the medication sheet and daily flow sheet. The diabetic record provides a log for review of the patient's response to the insulin regiments. It provides an overview where trends can be examined and adjustments made. When the patient goes home, they should be taught to keep a similar log for their personal use and for the physician to review.

## Insulin Syringes

Insulin requires a special syringe for proper measurement of the dosage. The syringe is a U-100 syringe to measure U-100 (100 units/mL) insulin. There are two types of U-100 insulin syringes, regular and low dose.

## U-100 Insulin Syringe

The U-100 insulin syringe is calibrated with the major markings at 10, 20, 30 etc. see picture below. Each small line is a **two unit** measure. To measure an odd numbered dose of insulin, such as 75 units, you need to measure the insulin between the 74 and 76 calibration.

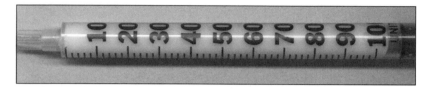

For greater than 50 units, use this U-100 syringe.

## U-100 Low Dosage Insulin Syringe

The low dosage insulin syringe is used to accurately measure low doses of insulin. It measures children's dosages and regular insulin dosages more accurately because the scale is calibrated for every unit. The syringe has an enlarged scale which is easier to read.

**Note:** *This low dosage syringe only measures up to 50 units of insulin or half as much as the standard syringe.*

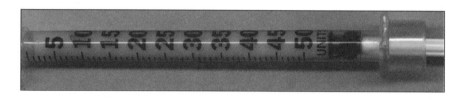

For less than 50 units use this low dose syringe.

**Note:** *Each small calibration line is one unit measure of insulin.*
**Note:** *Another low dosage syringe, not shown, measures up to 30 units of insulin or one third as much as the standard syringe.*

Administration of a correct dosage of insulin requires using the correct insulin with the correct insulin syringe and drawing up the prescribed number of units.

NPH, an intermediate acting insulin, is easily identified by the letter "N" on the bottle and Regular, a short acting insulin, is identifiable by the letter "R" on the bottle. Both types of insulin in this example are human U-100. All bottles come with an expiration date. This date should always be checked. Discard the bottle if it is past the expiration date.

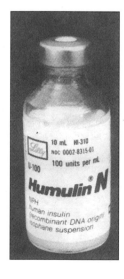
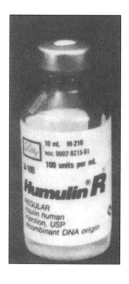

# Sliding Scale Regular Insulin

## Regular Insulin

Regular insulin is used for the immediate onset of activity and short duration of action. It is the only insulin that may be given intravenously and subcutaneously. It can be identified from its longer acting counterparts by its clear solution. Regular insulin is used frequently in the hospital setting for patients whose blood sugar is out of control for a variety of reasons. Some of these reasons are: dehydration and infection. Regular insulin is used frequently in these cases because of its immediate action and short duration.

Regular insulin may be given according to the sliding scale prescribed by the physician. The amount of insulin is related to the patient's finger stick blood sugar. The patient's blood sugar is checked by the nurse using a blood Glucose meter such as the Accucheck, Glucoscan, or Lifescan.

■ **Physician's Order:** Sliding Scale for Humulin Regular Insulin according to finger stick blood sugars q6h.

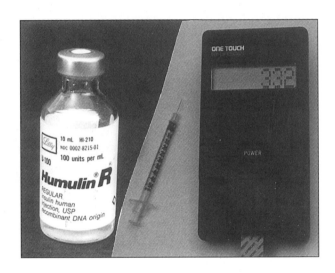

| Finger stick Blood Sugar Results (mg / dL) | | Regular Insulin Dosage |
|---|---|---|
| < 70 | _____ | call MD |
| 251 - 300 | _____ | 5 units Regular Insulin SQ |
| 301 - 350 | _____ | 10 units Regular Insulin SQ |
| 351 - 400 | _____ | 15 units Regular Insulin SQ |
| 401 - 500 | _____ | 20 units Regular Insulin SQ |
| >500 | _____ | call MD |

You have just checked your patient's 12 noon finger stick blood sugar and the One Touch reads a blood sugar of 332 mg / dL. How many units of Regular Insulin would you give?

Answer: 10 units

**Note:** *The above sliding scale is an example used on one patient. It is not a standard scale. Sliding scales are individualized for patients.*

■ **In summary, finger stick blood sugar is 332, mg/dL. Using this scale you would give 10 units of Regular Insulin.**

# Sliding Scale Insulin

Ms. Lu is a diabetic and has been admitted to the hospital with pneumonia. Her blood sugar has been out of control so the physician has ordered sliding scale insulin q6h.

Physician's order: Sliding Scale Regular Insulin

Finger Stick
Blood Sugar                                          Regular Insulin
(mg / dL)
<70 Call MD
201-250————————————————————4 units SQ
251-300————————————————————6 units SQ
301-350————————————————————8 units SQ
351-400————————————————————10 units SQ
410-450————————————————————12 units SQ
451-500————————————————————14 units SQ
>500—————————————————————call MD

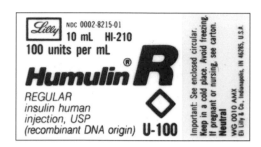

**Note:** *Shade the syringe where the top of the black plunger would be. The top of the plunger is the end nearest the needle. Check all shaded answers with another student just as if you were checking it with another nurse in a clinical setting.*

1.  At 0800 Ms. Lu's finger stick blood sugar is 364 mg /dL.
    Shade the insulin syringe with a pencil for the appropriate dosage.

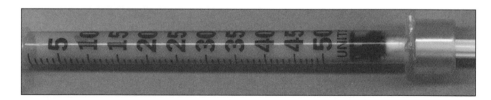

2.  At 1400 Ms. Lu's finger stick blood sugar is 310 mg /dL.
    Shade the insulin syringe for the appropriate dosage.

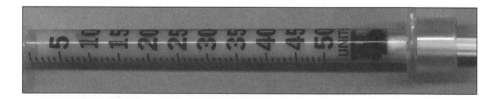

3.  At 2000 Ms. Lu's finger stick blood sugar is 253 mg /dL.
    Shade the insulin syringe for the appropriate dosage.

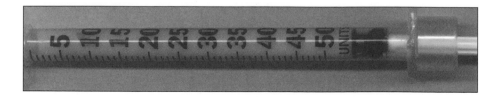

4. At 0200 Ms. Lu's finger stick blood sugar is 229 mg /dL.
   Shade the insulin syringe for the appropriate dosage.

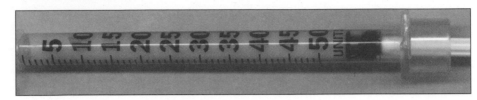

5. At 0800 Ms. Lu's finger stick blood sugar is 266 mg /dL.
   Shade the insulin syringe for the appropriate dosage.

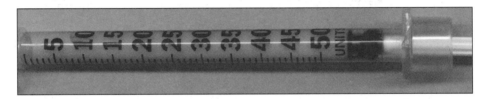

6. At 1400 Ms. Lu's finger stick blood sugar is 180 mg /dL.
   Shade the insulin syringe for the appropriate dosage.

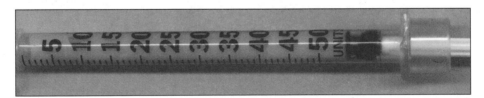

7. Ms. Beach has 32 units of humulin insulin 70/30 SQ ac breakfast ordered by her physician.

   Read the label and answer the following questions.

   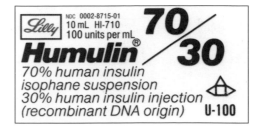

   a. What is the source of this insulin? _____

   b. Is this the correct source of insulin? _____

   c. What category of action is this insulin? _____

   d. Shade the U-100 insulin syringe to measure the correct dosage.

   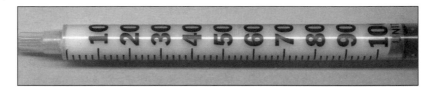

8. The physician has ordered 24 units of Humulin Insulin 70/30 SQ at 5 PM qd for Ms. Beach. Shade the U-100 insulin syringe to measure the correct dosage.

   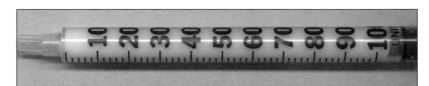

9. Mr. Johnson has been on Lantus insulin 42 units q HS for the last year. He has been admitted to the hospital. Physician orders to continue the Lantus 42 units SQ q HS

   Read the label and answer the following questions.

   a. What is the source of this insulin? _____

   b. Is this the correct source of insulin? _____

   c. What category of action is this insulin? _____

   d. Shade the U-100 insulin syringe to measure the correct dosage.

   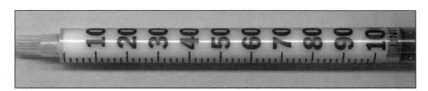

10. Mrs. Jones had an allergic reaction to the NPH Iletin 1 beef/pork insulin. The physician has changed the insulin to NPH Humulin Insulin 55 units SQ ac breakfast.

   Read the label and answer the following questions.

   a. What is the source of this insulin?  _____

   b. Is this the correct source of insulin?  _____

   c. What category of action is this insulin? _____

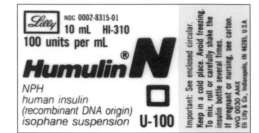

   d. Shade the U-100 insulin syringe to measure the correct dosage.

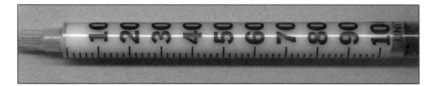

## Insulin given by a continuous infusion per electronic pump

See sample problem for heparin drips. Insulin uses the same formula to calculate the correct infusion rate. Remember only regular insulin may be given intravenously. When a patient is admitted for hyperglycemia and ketoacidosis, a bolus of regular insulin 0.1mg/kg may be given IV initally followed by an insulin infusion. The dosage for an insulin infusion is usually about 0.1 unit/kg/h.

11. Mrs. Simms, age fifty, with adult onset diabetes has been admitted to the emergency room with dehydration, hypotension, decreased level of consciousness and vomiting. She has not taken her Humulin NPH insulin because she has not been eating. Her blood sugar is checked and found to be 550 mg/dL. She weighs 165 lbs. The physician orders are to start an IV of 1000 mL of 0.45 Normal Saline followed by a bolus of **7 units of regular insulin IV push stat.**

   Read the label and answer the following questions.

   a. What is the source of this insulin?  _____

   b. Is this the correct source of insulin?  _____

   c. What category of action is this insulin?  _____

   d. Is the dosage appropriate for a 165 lb patient? _____

   e. Shade the U-50 insulin syringe to measure the correct dosage.

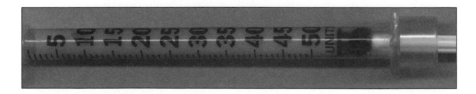

12. The physician orders an insulin drip for Mrs. Simms to run at 7 units per hour. Mrs. Simms weighs 165 lbs.

    The label reads 50 units of regular insulin in 50 mL of NS.

    a.  Is this dosage of insulin reasonable? _____

    b.  The insulin is infused by pump. Calculate the flow rate in mL/h. _____

13. Mr. Swanson is a large man weighing 250 pounds. His finger stick blood sugar is 400. An insulin drip is ordered at 11 units per hour.

    The label reads 75 units of regular insulin in 100 mL of NS.

    a.  Is this dosage of insulin reasonable? _____

    b.  The insulin is infused by pump. Calculate the flow rate in mL/h. _____

14. The physician orders an insulin drip at 8 units an hour. Mr. Blair's last finger stick blood sugar was 250 mg/dL. Mr. Blair weighs 175 pounds.

    The label reads 100 units of regular insulin in 100 mL of NS.

    a.  Is this dosage of insulin reasonable? _____

    b.  The insulin is infused by pump. Calculate the flow rate in mL/h. _____

15. Mrs. Schultz's blood sugar is 300 mg/dL. She weighs 110 pounds. The physician has ordered an insulin drip at 5 units per hour.

    The label reads 50 units of regular insulin in 100 mL of NS.

    a.  Is this dosage of insulin reasonable? _____

    b.  The insulin is infused by pump. Calculate the flow rate in mL/h. _____

# Measuring two types of insulin in the same syringe

The 1993 Diabetes Control and Complications Trials (DCCT) showed that the complications of diabetes were significantly reduced by tighter control of the blood sugar. Retinopathy was reduced by 76%, kidney disease by 35%, and neuropathy by 60%. This study was conducted with diabetes type 1 patients. Recent studies also show that diabetes type 2 clients also benefit from tighter control of blood sugars.

The number of diabetics using flexible insulin therapy, which includes either multiple daily injections or insulin pumps, has increased dramatically since the release of DCCT results.

The base line need for insulin is met by giving NPH, Lente or Ultalente once or twice a day and then Regular or Humalog insulin to match the carbohydrates of each meal.

Rather than give two injections of insulin, the NPH and regular are drawn into one syringe. This reduces the number of injections the patient will receive. The illustrations depict how the two dosages are mixed to give one injection.

For this patient the physician has ordered **25 units of NPH insulin** and **5 units of regular insulin** for the 4 PM dosage.

The photographs show how to measure each dosage in the correct sequence.

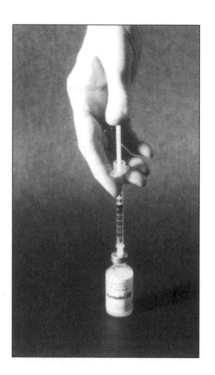

### Step 1

Inject 25 units of air into the bottle of NPH.
This will prevent a vacuum from occurring.

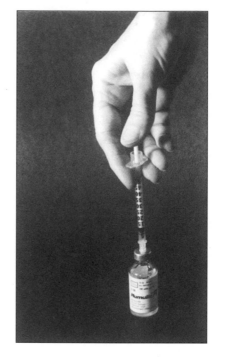

### Step 2

Inject 5 units of air into the bottle of regular insulin.

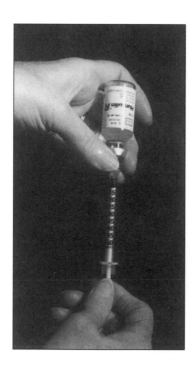

### Step 3

Turn the bottle upside down and withdraw 5 units of regular insulin.

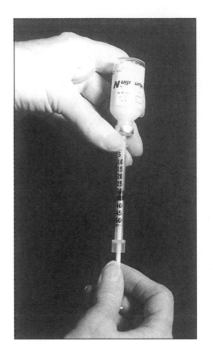

**Step 4**

Turn the NPH bottle upside down and insert the needle into the NPH bottle, **being careful not to inject any of the 5 units** of regular insulin. With the bottle upside down, **withdraw 25 units** of NPH. The two insulins together will be at the **30 unit** marker of the syringe.

> Note: *Before drawing up the NPH insulin gently roll the bottle to mix. Do not shake. Shaking can break down the particles as well as causing bubbles.*

This sequence is extremely important. The regular insulin should be drawn up first, because if a drop of regular insulin goes into the NPH bottle no harm is done. However, if the NPH should go into the regular insulin, the regular insulin would be tainted and have to be discarded.

These steps will be useful to the patient or nurse in measuring the correct dosage.

**Helpful Hint**

**To help you remember the sequence:**

> **F**ast **F**irst (Regular Insulin)
> **S**low **S**econd (NPH)

Note: *Many medical centers require double signatures on the MAR for insulin. Have another nurse check the order, the amount in the syringe for both dosages, along with expiration date on the bottle and then cosign the MAR.*

16. The physician ordered NPH insulin 22 units SQ and regular insulin 11 units SQ ac breakfast. Draw an arrow on the syringe indicating first the regular insulin and then the NPH insulin.

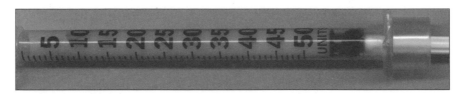

17. The physican ordered NPH insulin 14 units SQ and regular insulin 8 units SQ ac dinner. Draw an arrow on the syringe indicating the regular insulin and then the NPH insulin.

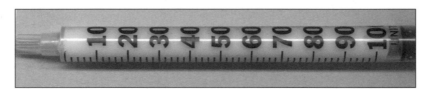

18. The physican ordered NPH insulin 16 units SQ and regular insulin 8 units SQ ac breakfast. Draw an arrow on the syringe indicating the regular insulin and then the NPH insulin.

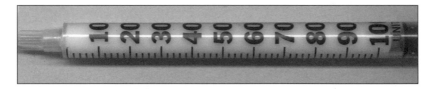

19. The physican ordered NPH insulin 16 units SQ and regular insulin 7 units SQ ac dinner. Draw an arrow on the syringe indicating the regular insulin and then the NPH insulin.

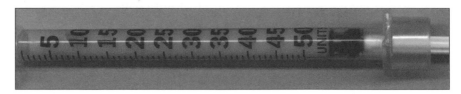

20. The physican ordered NPH insulin 20 units SQ and regular insulin 14 units SQ ac breakfast. Draw an arrow on the syringe indicating the regular insulin and then the NPH insulin.

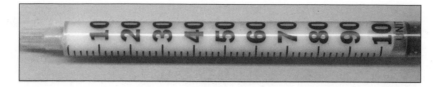

Answers: Chapter 10, 1-20

1. 10 units
2. 8 units
3. 6 units
4. 4 units
5. 6 units
6. none
7. a. Human insulin
   b. Yes. Patient has been on human
   c. NPH Intermediate acting insulin and Regular short acting
   d. 32 marker
8. 24 marker
9. a. human
   b. Yes. Patient has been on Lantus
   c. Long acting
   d. 42 marker
10. a. Human insulin
    b. Yes, order was changed to human
    c. Intermediate
    d. 55 unit marker

11. a. Human
    b. Yes. She has been on human NPH
    c. Short action
    d. Yes
    e. 7 unit marker
12. a. Yes
    b. 7 mL/h
13. a. Yes
    b. 15 mL/h
14. a. Yes
    b. 8 mL/h
15. a. Yes
    b. 10 mL/h
16. 11 unit marker for regular and 33 unit marker for NPH
17. 8 unit marker for regular and 22 unit marker for NPH
18. 8 unit marker for regular and 24 unit marker for NPH
19. 7 unit marker for regular and 23 unit marker for NPH
20. 14 unit marker for regular and 34 unit marker for NPH

# 11

## Chapter Eleven

# Titrated Drugs used in Critical Care

# Titrated Drugs Used in Critical Care

## Introduction

The content in Chapter Eleven may not be required as a part of the nursing curriculum. However, it is included as a reference for nurses working in specialty areas.

Included in this chapter: Hints for safe IV drug calculation, using the infusion pump to titrate potent vasopressor drugs, sample problems and practice problems.

**Hints for safe IV drug calculations using titrated drips**

1. Always use an electronic infusion pump to deliver titrated drugs.
2. Obtain an accurate weight of your patient.
3. Use a calculator
4. Count zeros carefully and place decimal points accurately. An error in the placement of the decimal point can be disastrous to the patient.
5. Double check the dosage with another RN. Always double check the results. Ask another RN to also calculate the problem.
6. Always check the concentration of the drug that is hanging before doing your calculations.
7. Label all lines and all infusion pumps with the drug that is infusing. Frequently critically ill patients are on multiple drips which can become tangled. These lines need to be untangled and carefully labeled. Be especially careful not to confuse the tube feeding line with the intravenous lines. Lipids and oral tubing feeding look very similar lying side by side on the bed. Also label the front of the pump with the name of the drug when there are several drips running at once. This makes it easy to identify the drip when you want to change the infusion rate.

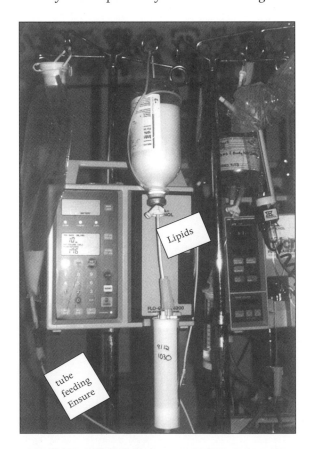

## Critical Care Chart

The chart below identifies medications that are ordered in different ways. The four categories are **mg/min**, **mcg/min**, **units/min**, and **mcg/kg/min**. Different institutions may have variations of the concentrations of the drugs on the chart. The formulas in this chapter will allow you to figure the correct dosage regardless of how the drug is mixed. However, if you are mixing your own medications the concentration columns will provide a guideline. The maintenance dosage column provides a guideline for the therapeutic range of the drug. It is best to titrate the medications within the maintenance range, but at times it is necessary to know the maximum amount that may be given.

### Critical Care Drug Chart

| Drug | Maintenance | Maximum | Concentration | Conc. /ml |
|------|-------------|---------|---------------|-----------|
| DRUGS ORDERED IN **MG/MIN** | | | | |
| bretylium (Bretylol) | 1-2 mg/min | 2 mg/min | 2 g /250 mL D5W | 8 mg/mL |
| lidocaine (Xylocaine) | 1-4 mg/min | 4 mg/min | 2 g /250 mL D5W | 8 mg/mL |
| procainamide (Pronestyl) | 2-6 mg/min | 6 mg/min | 2 g 250 mL D5W | 8 mg/mL |
| | | | | |
| DRUGS ORDERED IN **MCG/MIN** | | | | |
| epinephrine (Adrenaline) | 1-4 mcg/min | 4 mcg/min | 2 mg/250 mL D5W | 8 mcg/mL |
| isoproterenol (Isuprel) | 0.5-5 mcg/min | 30 mcg/min | 2 mg/250 mL D5W | 8 mcg/mL |
| nitroglycerin (Tridil) | 5-400 mcg/min | 400 mcg/min | 50 mg/250 mL D5W | 200 mcg/mL |
| norepinephrine (Levophed) | 2-4 mcg/min | 47 mcg/min | 4 mg/250 mL D5W | 16 mcg/mL |
| phenylephrine (Neo-Synephrine) | 40-60 mcg/min | 180 mcg/min | 10 mg/250 mL D5W | 40 mcg/mL |
| | | | | |
| DRUGS ORDERED IN **UNITS/MIN** | | | | |
| vasopressin (Pitressin) | 0.1-0.9 u/min | 0.9 u/min | 150 u/150 mL D5W | 1 u/mL |
| | | | | |
| DRUGS ORDERED IN **MCG/KG/MIN** | | | | |
| amrinone (Inocor) | 5-10 mcg/kg/min | 12 mcg/kg/min | 100 mg/100 mL NS | 1000 mcg/mL |
| dobutamine (Dobutrex) | 2.5-10 mcg/kg/min | 40 mcg/kg/min | 500 mg/250 mL D5W | 2000 mcg/mL |
| dopamine ( Intropin) | 1-20 mcg/kg/min | 50 mcg/kg/min | 400 mg/250 mL D5W | 1600 mcg/mL |
| esmolol (Brevibloc) | 50-200 mcg/kg/min | 300 mcg/kg/min | 5 Gm/500 mL D5W | 10000 mcgmL |
| nitroprusside (Nipride) | 0.5-10 mcg/kg/m | 10 mcg/kg/min | 50 mg/250 mL D5W | 200 mcg/mL |

**Note:** *Many of the drugs come premixed by the pharmaceutical companies. Your hospital may not order the drugs in the above concentrations. If you have to mix the drugs listed on the chart, this is an acceptable way of mixing them.*

# Milligrams per minute

Some drugs are ordered in milligrams (mg) per minute (min). This requires an infusion pump to deliver a precise dosage.

**Formula: Milligrams/min**

$$\frac{\text{Concentration/mL x infusion rate (IR)}}{60 \text{ min/h}} = \text{Dose/min}$$

Example:

A lidocaine drip is running at 45 mL/h. The concentration is 4 mg/mL. How many mg/min is the patient receiving?

$$\frac{4 \text{ mg/mL } \times 45 \text{ mL/h}}{60 \text{ min/h}} = \frac{180}{60} = 3 \text{ mg/min}$$

■ **In summary, lidocaine 45 mL/h = 3 mg/min.**

# Infusion Rate in mL/h

This formula may be used to calculate any drug for which the dose is ordered per minute.

**Formula: Infusion Rate in mL / h**

$$\frac{\text{Desired Dose / min x 60 min / h}}{\text{Concentration / mL}} = \text{IR in mL/h.}$$

Example:

The physician orders lidocaine 3 mg / minute. Concentration 4 mg / mL.

$$\frac{3 \text{ mg} \times 60 \text{ mL/h}}{4 \text{ mg/mL}} = \frac{180}{4} = 45 \text{ mL/h}$$

■ **In summary, lidocaine 3 mg / min = 45 mL/h**

# Lidocaine

Lidocaine indications: ventricular dysrhythmias especially premature ventricular contraction (PVC's).
Maintenance Range is 1-4 mg per minute.
Lidocaine is a drug that is prescribed in mg per min. It is usually mixed in 2 different concentrations.

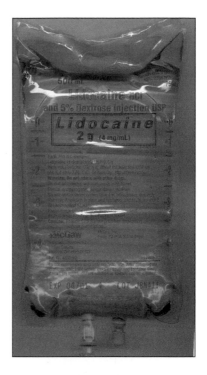

**Lidocaine Standard Concentration Table**
Standard solution lidocaine 2 g in 500 mL of D5W or 4 mg/mL

> 4 mg / min = 60 mL/h
> 3 mg / min = 45 mL/h
> 2 mg / min = 30 mL/h
> 1 mg / min = 15 mL/h

The physician orders 2 mg per min.
What is the infusion rate? _____
Use the Standard Concentration table for the answer.

Answer: 30 mL/h

If the physician orders 3 mg / min, how many
mL/h would you run the IV? _____

Answer: 45 mL/h

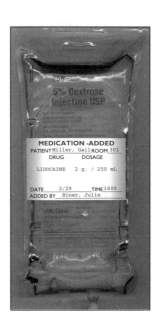

**Lidocaine Double Concentration Table**
Double Concentrated Solution of Lidocaine *2 G
Lidocaine in 250 mL D 5 W or 8 mg/mL.

> 4 mg / min = 30 mL/h
> 3 mg / min = 22 mL/h
> 2 mg / min = 15 mL/h
> 1 mg / min = 7 mL/h

*Used with patients on fluid restrictions

If the physician orders 2 mg per minute and you have a double
concentrated solution, what is the infusion rate? _____
Use the Double Concentration Table for the answer.

Answer: 15 mL/h

If the physician orders 3 mg / min, what is the infusion rate?_____
Use the Double Concentration table for the answer.

Answer: 22 mL/h

# Micrograms Per mL

**nitroglycerin**

Indications:  control chest pain with stable and unstable angina
congestive heart failure
coronary vasospasm

Initial infusion rate 5-10 mcg / min
Maintenance infusion rate 5-400 mcg / min

Read the label for the concentration of nitroglycerin

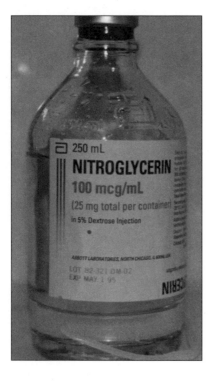

**Note:** *Nitroglycerin must be mixed in a glass bottle rather than a plastic bag to prevent absorption of the drug into the plastic. A special non PVC plastic tubing without a filter should be used with a glass bottle.*

**Formula: mcg / mL**

$$\frac{\text{known amount of drug (D)}}{\text{total volume of diluent (V)}} = \text{amount of drug per mL}$$

1 mg = 1,000 mcg
25 mg x 1000 = 25,000 mcg

$$\frac{25,000 \text{ mcg}}{250 \text{ mL}} = 100 \text{ mcg / mL}$$

In summary, 25 mg of nitroglycerin diluted in 250 mL of D5W gives a concentration of 100 mcg/mL.

# Micrograms Per Minute

A nitroglycerin drip is running at 3 mL/h. The concentration of nitroglycerin is 100 mcg/mL. How many mcg/minute is the patient receiving?

**Formula: mcg / min**

$$\frac{\text{Concentration /mL x infusion rate (mL/h)}}{60 \text{ min / h}} = \text{dose / minute}$$

$$\frac{100 \text{ mcg/mL x 3 mL/h}}{60 \text{ min/h}} = 5 \text{ mcg / min}$$

Answer: 5 mcg / min

In summary, an infusion rate of 3 mL per hour = 5 mcg per min.

# Infusion Rate in Milliliters Per Hour

In the previous sample problem, you were asked to determine the dose per minute. You were given the infusion rate. In this problem you will be asked to determine the infusion rate. You are given the dose / min.

The physician orders nitroglycerin 5 mcg / min.

**Formula: Infusion Rate**

$$\frac{\text{Desired Dose /min x 60 min/h}}{\text{Concentration / mL}} = \text{Infusion Rate in mL / h}$$

Example:

$$\frac{5 \text{ mcg/min x 60 min/h}}{100 \text{ mcg / mL}} = \frac{300}{100} = 3 \text{ mL/h}$$

In summary, nitroglycerin 5 mcg / min = an infusion rate of 3 mL/h.

# Micrograms Per Minute

Mr. Rankin is having chest pain. The physician has ordered a nitroglycerin drip. Titrate until the chest pain is controlled. Start nitroglycerin drip at 10 mcg/min.

Read the label

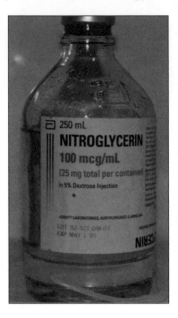

1.  The nitroglycerin drip is to start at 10 mcg / min.

    Give? _____ mL / h.

    **Formula:** $\dfrac{\text{Desired dose/ min x 60 mL/h}}{\text{Concentration/mL}} = \text{IR mL/h}$

2.  The nitroglycerin drip has now been titrated up to 12 mL/h.

    How many mcg/min is Mr. Rankin receiving? _____

    **Formula:** $\dfrac{\text{Concentration per mL x infusion rate}}{60 \text{ min}} = \text{Dose/min.}$

3.  The nitroglycerin drip is at 15 mL/h.

    How many mcg/min is Mr. Rankin receiving? _____

4.  The nitroglycerin drip is at 18 mL/h.

    How many mcg/min is Mr. Rankin receiving? _____

5.  Mr. Rankin is now comfortable with no chest pain. The nurse from the previous shift has left the nitroglycerin drip at 25 mL/h for the last 2 hours.

    How many mcg/min is Mr. Rankin receiving? _____

# Micrograms / Kilogram / Minute

mcg / kg / min
Concentration Factor

▮ The physician orders: Titrate the nitroprusside (Nipride) to keep the blood pressure less than 140 mm Hg systolic. The patient weighs 124 lbs or 56 kg.

Read the drug label.

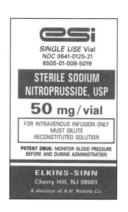

The next two problems use the same nitroprusside concentration.

Nitoprusside 50 mg / 250 mL of D5W =  200 mcg / mL

Concentration = 200 mcg / mL

Determine the concentration factor for this patient weighing 56 kg and the nitroprusside concentration at 200 mcg / mL.

---

Formula: concentration factor for mcg/kg/min.

$$\frac{\dfrac{\text{mcg/mL}}{\text{kg}}}{60 \text{ min}} = \text{Concentration Factor} \quad \text{or} \quad \frac{\text{mcg}}{\text{mL}} \bigg/ \text{kg} \bigg/ 60 \text{ min} = \text{concentration factor}$$

$$\frac{200 \text{ mcg/mL}}{56 \text{ kg}} = 3.57 \qquad \frac{3.57}{60 \text{ min}} = 0.059$$

Concentration factor    0.059    Save this number.

---

**Note:** *The concentration factor of 0.059 can be used over and over again to quickly recalculate the number of microgram/kilogram/minute this patient is receiving.*

# mcg / kg / min Using Concentration Factor
# With the Infusion Rate Given.

If the IV is running at 20 mL per hour, determine the number of mcg/kg/min the patient is receiving using the concentration factor of 0.059. (nitroprusside from previous problem)

Formula: Mcg/kg/min

Concentration factor x mL / h = mcg/kg/min

0.059 x 20 = 1.18 or 1.2

Answer: 1.2 mcg/kg/min

■ In summary, 20 mL / h = 1.2 mcg / kg / min.
The proper way to chart the nitroprusside is to use both mcg/kg/min rather than just mL / h.

# Infusion Rate Using the Concentration Factor
# With mcg / kg / min Given.

■ The physician orders nitroprusside 3 mcg/kg/min.

Formula: Infusion Rate

$$\frac{mcg/kg/min}{concentration\ factor} = Infusion\ Rate\ mL / h$$

$$\frac{3\ mcg/kg/min}{0.059} = 50.8\ or\ 51\ mL / h$$

■ In summary, 3 mcg/kg/min = 51 mL / h for the IV rate.

# mcg / kg / min for nitroprusside

> **Nitroprusside (Nipride)**
> **Note:** *Nitroprusside is a potent vasodilator that acts within 30-60 seconds to lower the blood pressure. Protect Nipride from light by wrapping it in aluminum foil or a non transparent plastic bag provided by the manufacturer.*
>
> nitroprusside dose information:
> Maintenance infusion rate is 0.5-10 mcg/kg/min.
> Thiocynate level is recommended to prevent toxicity from prolonged use.

6. The physician orders titrate nitroprusside to keep Mr. Reyes systolic blood pressure below 140 mm Hg. Mr. Reyes weighs 160 lbs. The IV is running at 8 mL / h. Read the label to determine the concentration of the drug.

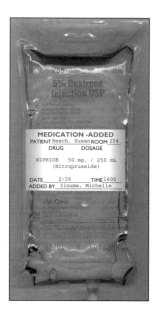

a. What is Mr. Reyes weight in kg.?  _____

Formula: $\dfrac{\text{pounds}}{2.2}$ = kg

b. How many mcg/mL?  _____

Formula: $\dfrac{\text{Known amount of drug (D)}}{\text{Total volume of diluent (V)}}$ = Amount of drug / mL

c. What is the concentration factor?  _____

Formula: $\dfrac{\frac{\text{mcg/mL}}{\text{Weight (kg)}}}{60 \text{ min.}}$ = Concentration factor

d. How many mcg/kg/min is Mr. Reyes receiving? _____

Formula: Concentration factor x mL/h = mcg/kg/min

7.  Mr. Reyes BP is 150 mm Hg systolic and the RN has increased the nitroprusside to 13 mL/h. Use the concentration factor.
    How many mcg/kg/min is Mr. Reyes receiving? _____

8.  Mr. Reyes BP is 145 mm Hg systolic and the RN has increased the nitroprusside to 22 mL/h. Use the concentration factor.
    How many mcg/kg/min is Mr. Reyes receiving? _____

9.  Mr. Reyes is restless and the systolic BP is still at 145-150 mm Hg. The nitroprusside is now at 44 mL/h. Use the concentration factor.
    How many mcg/kg/min is Mr Reyes receiving? _____

10. Mr. Reyes is more relaxed and the systolic BP is 110 mm Hg. The nitroprusside has been gradually reduced to 10 mL / h. Use the concentration factor.
    How many mcg/kg/min is Mr. Reyes receiving? _____

# Dopamine

Dopamine's action raises the systolic blood pressure and dilates the renal vascular beds improving urinary output. It is used to maintain a systolic blood pressure of greater than 90 mmHg. Its effect is dose related as demonstrated in the chart on the next page. Dopamine should not be used to support the blood pressure, without first ensuring that adequate fluid resuscitation has occurred. Fluids are the first line of defense with hypovolemic shock. Dopamine is used to maintain the blood pressure when fluids have failed to increase the blood pressure adequately. Dopamine is also used for cardiogenic shock.
Maintenance dosage is 1-20 mcg/kg/min.
Maximum dosage: rarely greater than 50 mcg/kg/min.

**Note:** *Dopamine is inactivated by alkaline solutions. Never push sodium bicarbonate through a dopamine line.*

# Dopamine *cont.*

The chart shows the dose related effects of dopamine.

**Lower range** of 0.5 to 2 mcg/kg/min, dopamine causes vasodilation of the renal vascular beds which is accompanied by increased glomerular filtration rate, renal blood low, and urinary output. When it is used for renal perfusion, the rate of administration is from 0.5-2 mcg/kg/min. The urinary output must be monitored carefully.

**Intermediate range** of 2-10 mcg/kg/min, dopamine stimulates the beta 1 adrenoceptors and causes an increase in cardiac output, stroke volume, myocardial contractility, and renal blood flow. When dopamine is used to support a systolic blood pressure greater than 90 mmHg it is usually started at 5 mcg/kg/min and titrated up or down according to the patient's response.

**Higher range** of 10-20 mcg/kg/min, dopamine has some effect on alpha adrenoceptors, which will continue to raise the blood pressure, but also start to produce vasoconstriction of the skeletal muscle vascular beds. When dopamine is infused at rates greater than 20 mcg/kg/min, the incidence of increased systemic vascular resistance, myocardial oxygen consumption, tachyarrhythmias, and decreased urinary output are very high.

## Dopamine (Intropin) dosage phenomena

| | Renal & Lower Range | Intermediate Range | Higher Range |
|---|---|---|---|
| The Effects of Intropin at 3 Dose Ranges | 0.5-2 mcg/kg/min | 2-10 mcg/kg/min | 10- 20 mcg/kg/min |
| Cardiac Output | no change | increase | increase |
| Stroke Volume | no change | increase | increase |
| Heart Rate | no change | there is an initial increase followed by a decrease towards normal rates as infusion continues | increase |
| Myocardial Contractility | no change | increase | increase |
| Potential for Excessive Myocardial Oxygen Demands | *low coronary blood flow increased | *low coronary blood increase | data unavailable |
| Potential for Tachyarrhythmias | *low | *low | moderate |
| Total Systemic Resistance | slight decrease to no change | no change to slight increase | increase |
| Renal Blood Flow | increase | increase | decrease |
| Urine Output | increase | increase | decrease |

* Low but monitor parameter carefully

# mcg/kg/min Dopamine

In the following problems the nurse has adjusted the infusion rate according to the clinical response of the patient. When the infusion rate is changed, the dosage must be recalculated in mcg/kg/min.

11. The physician orders: Titrate dopamine to keep Mrs. Jackson's systolic blood pressure greater than 90 mm Hg. Mrs. Jackson weighs 150 lbs. The dopamine is running at 5 mL / h.
    Read the label for the concentration of Dopamine.

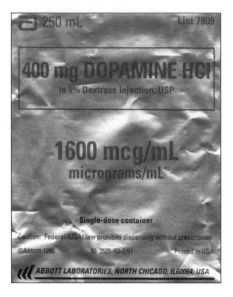

  a. What is Mrs. Jackson's weight in Kg.?  _____

     **Formula:** $\dfrac{\text{pounds}}{2.2} = \text{kg}$

  b. How many mcg/mL?  _____

     **Formula:** $\dfrac{\text{Known amount of drug (D)}}{\text{Total volume of diluent (V)}} = \text{Amount of drug / mL}$

  c. What is the concentration factor? _____ Save this answer for the next few problems.

     **Formula:** $\dfrac{\frac{\text{mcg/mL}}{\text{Weight(kg)}}}{60 \text{ min.}} = \text{Concentration factor}$

  d. How many mcg/kg/min is Mrs. Jackson receiving? _____

     **Formula:** Concentration factor x mL/h = mcg/kg/min

12. Mrs. Jackson's systolic blood pressure is 85 mm Hg. The nurse has increased the dopamine rate to 12 mL/h. Use the concentration factor.
    How many mcg/kg/min is Mrs. Jackson receiving?  _____

13. The dopamine on Mrs. Jackson is now running at 43 mL/h. Use the concentration factor.
    How many mcg/kg/min is Mrs. Jackson receiving?  _____

14. Mrs. Jackson's BP has been running 128 mm Hg systolic. The dopamine has been reduced to 35 mL/h. Use the concentration factor.
    How many mcg/kg/min is Mrs. Jackson receiving?  _____

# mcg/kg/min Dobutamine

## Dobutamine (Dobutrex)

Indications: Used for its inotropic effect on depressed cardiac contractility. Used in patients with cardiogenic shock and congestive heart failure. Onset of action is 1-2 min; duration of action 10 min.
Maintenance infusion range: 2.5 mcg/kg/min —10 mcg/kg/min
Maximum dosage: 40 mcg/kg/min

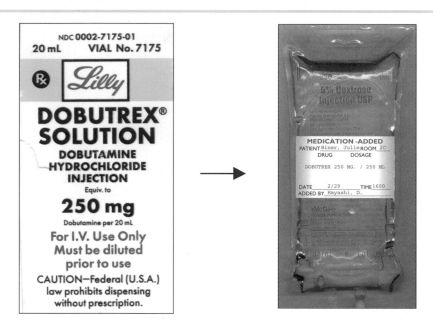

15. The physician orders dobutamine 3 mcg/kg/min for Mrs. Gonzales who weighs 141 lbs.

   a.   What is Mrs. Gonzales weight in kg.? _____

   Formula: $\dfrac{pounds}{2.2}$ = kg

   b.   How many mcg/mL?                    _____

   Formula: $\dfrac{\text{Known amount of drug (D)}}{\text{Total volume of diluent (V)}}$ = Amount of drug / mL

   c.   What is the concentration factor?    _____

   Formula: $\dfrac{\frac{mcg/mL}{Weight (kg)}}{60 min.}$ = Concentration factor

   d.   How many mL/h?                      _____

   Formula: $\dfrac{mcg/kg/min}{\text{Concentration Factor}}$ = Infusion Rate

16. The physician increases the dobutamine on Mrs. Gonzales to 5 mcg/kg/min.
    How many mL/h should she receive?         _____

17. The physician increases the dobutamine on Mrs. Gonzales to 7 mcg/kg/min.
    How many mL/h should she receive?         _____

18. The physician increases the dobutamine on Mrs. Gonzales to 10 mcg/kg/min.
    How many mL/h should she receive?                   _____

19. The physician orders dobutamine 2.5 mcg/kg/min for Mr. Paczic who weighs 193 lbs.
    Dobutamine 250 mg in 250 mL D5W.

    a.   What is Mr. Paczic's weight in Kg?              _____

         **Formula:** $\frac{pounds}{2.2}$ = kg

    b.   How many mcg of dobutamine per mL?             _____

         **Formula:** $\frac{\text{Known amount of drug (D)}}{\text{Total volume of diluent (V)}}$ = Amount of drug / mL

    c.   What is the concentration factor?              _____

         **Formula:** $\frac{\frac{\text{Mcg/mL}}{\text{Weigh(kg)}}}{60 \text{ min.}}$ = Concentration factor

    d.   How many mL per hour?                          _____

         **Formula:** $\frac{\text{mcg/kg/min}}{\text{Concentration Factor}}$ = Infusion Rate

20. The physician increases the dobutamine to 3 mcg/kg/min on Mr. Paczic.
    How many mL/h should he receive?                    _____

21. The physician increases the dobutamine to 4.5 mcg/kg/min on Mr. Paczic.
    How many mL/h should he receive?                    _____

22. The physician increases the dobutamine rate to 32 mL/h.
    How many mcg/kg/min is Mr. Paczic receiving?        _____

23. The nurse increases the dobutamine rate to 34 mL/h.
    How many mcg/kg/min is Mr. Paczic receiving?        _____

Answers: Chapter 11, 1-23

1.  6 mL / h
2.  20 mcg/min
3.  25 mcg/min
4.  30 mcg/min
5.  42 mcg/min
6.  a. 72.7 kg  b. 200 mcg/mL
    c. 0.046  d. 0.4 mcg/kg/min.
7.  0.598 or 0.6 mcg/kg/min
8.  1 mcg/kg/min
9.  2 mcg/kg/min
10. 0.46 or 0.5 mcg/kg/min
11. a. 68 kg  b. 1600 mcg/mL
    c. 0.39 or 0.4  d. 2 mcg/kg/min
12. 4.6 mcg/kg/min or 5 mcg/kg/min

13. 17 mcg/kg/min
14  14 mcg/kg/min
15. a. 64 kg b. 1000 mcg/mL
    c. 0.26  d. 11.5 or 12 mL
16. 19 mL / h
17. 26.9 or 27 mL / h
18. 38 mL / h
19. a. 87.7 kg  b. 1000 mcg/mL
    c. 0.19  d. 13 mL / h
20. 16 mL / h
21. 24 mL / h
22. 6 mcg / kg / min
23. 6.5 mcg / kg / min

# 12

## Chapter Twelve

# Community Nursing and the Elderly

# The Elderly

## Background Information

Employment opportunities for nurses in the home care setting and community will be plentiful in the coming years with the baby boomers aging and the proliferation of managed care. Nurses are in a key position to help the community and especially the elderly use their medications safely and correctly. The home health nurse forms part of the interdisciplinary team caring for clients in the community. The nurse collaborates with the pharmacist and other health care professionals involved with the care of the patient. The pharmacist can be an invaluable resource for providing information and expertise.

Patients will receive drug therapy at home which in the past was done only in the hospital. Some examples of this are IV antibiotics, IV chemotherapy, and IV vasopressors. The patient may be started on the drug in the hospital to be observed closely for signs and symptoms of adverse drug reactions. When stabilized, the patient will be sent home to continue the drug therapy. In the past, the patient remained in the hospital until the drug therapy was completed. In the home setting, the home care service helps the patient become comfortable with the treatment regime. The insurance may cover a predetermined number of visits by the RN and then periodically thereafter. Therefore, the nurse needs to teach the patient or family members to administer the care after the initial visits. In the case of IV antibiotics the family may actually hang the IV PB medications and also learn to set the infusion pump and care for the IV site. The nurse's teaching skills become paramount in ensuring that the patient and family can carry on with the prescribed regime.

## Patient Education for "Over the Counter Drugs"

Several drugs such as Pepcid and Tagamet are sold over the counter and others may soon be approved. Previously, the patient could only obtain these drugs by seeing a physician and obtaining a prescription. Now these drugs can be obtained by anyone from the local pharmacy or major drugstore chain. The patients will need education regarding how to use these drugs appropriately. Nurses and pharmacists will play an increasingly significant role in patient education of "over the counter drugs".

## Proliferation of New Drugs on the Market

Nurses will need to keep abreast of new drugs and drug therapy. Use of robotics and computers by the pharmaceutical industry has already decreased the time it takes to develop new drugs. The Federal Drug Administration has streamlined the approval process of these new drugs, and increased advertising by pharmaceutical companies has made consumers aware of many of the new medications on the market.

## Drugs and the Elderly

The elderly population is increasing. Eighty six percent of the elderly have chronic health problems requiring four or more prescription drugs on a regular basis. The incident of adverse drug reactions is very high in this age bracket. An adverse drug reaction (ADR) is defined as an unwanted response to a drug. Polypharmacy, which means a patient is on too many drugs, is very common. The patient may be seeing several doctors who are unaware of drugs or treatments that the other physicians have prescribed. A study, undertaken at the University of Manchester, England, by Lindley, Tully, Paramsothy and Tallis, reported in the journal *Age and Aging* 1992; 21: 294-300 on the relationship of inappropriate medication prescribing and adverse drug reactions in the elderly. One hundred and seventy-five drugs were discontinued on or shortly after admission of 113 patients because they were deemed to be unnecessary. One hundred and three patients experienced 151 ARDS. Seventy five ARDS were as a result of contraindications or inappropriate prescribing. The homecare nurse is often the one who identifies polypharmacy and/or adverse drug reactions. He/she can confer with the physicians involved to alleviate the situation.

## Essentials in Patient Teaching

1. Obtain a complete medication history which includes prescription drugs, over the counter drugs, vitamins and herbal medications. Herbal medicines have become very popular in recent years. The following are some of the items found on the shelf at the local health food store—Chamomile, Echinacea, Flax, Garlic, Ginger, Ginkgo, Ginseng, Kava, and St. John's Wort. Many patients believe in this form of alternative therapy and may want to continue taking herbal remedies. For example, St. John's Wort may be beneficial for depression. It is used more frequently in Europe and it is regulated as a drug. In the United States it is not regulated and it is sold as a health food and herbal supplement. In the Internet-Enhanced Journal of Pharmacology and Therapeutics, Dr. David J. Kroll writes, "In the United States, the Dietary Supplement Health and Education Act (DSHEA) of 1994 allows herbs to be sold legally as long as no claims for disease treatment are made on the product label.... The DSHEA has no require- 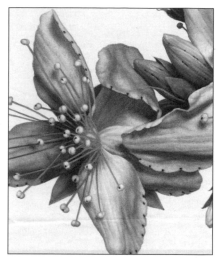 ment for product standardization of any pharmacologically active principle, demonstration of bioavailability or efficacy, or safety assessment when the product is used either alone or in combination with prescription or over-the counter drugs." The community health nurse accommodates to the client's health care practices, and as long as the herbal remedy is not harmful, integrates the herbal medicine into the care plan. Just like other drugs, this information should be included in the medication history. Drug interactions and incompatibilities should also be taken into account. For example, St. John's Wort should not be taken concurrently with other antidepressants, and it can also cause photosensitivity. Specific information on herbal medicines can be found in recently published books. Another example for the necessity of specifically asking about over the counter drugs is illustrated by coronary artery bypass surgery patients. Some may take aspirin regularly for arthritic pain. In one instance, when a patient was asked what medications were currently being taken, a detailed list of prescription medications was given. However, the patient who had taken aspirin, had excessive bleeding from the chest tubes. The patient did not think it was important enough to mention, as it was just an over the counter drug. Aspirin affects the platelets and can cause post operative bleeding.

2. Identify all known medication allergies and label the chart and medication records in appropriate places.

3. Write down for the patient and family both the generic and brand name of the drug.

4. Encourage the patient and the family to identify the drug by the name and not the color and size of the pill.

5. Help the patient and the family understand the purpose and action of the drug.

6. Determine how the drug should be taken in relationship to meals.

7. Advise the patient of any precautions to be taken concerning driving or operating machinery.

8. Identify drugs that may cause adverse reactions with alcohol consumption.

9. Encourage the patient to use one pharmacy to fill prescriptions. This allows the pharmacist to monitor all the patient's medications and identify any incompatibilities.

10. Teach the home care patients to store current medications separately from noncurrent drugs. Patients may have many drugs stored in their medicine cabinet. Drugs are sometimes started, discontinued and started again by the physician for various reasons. For safety practices, store current drugs and discontinued drugs separately. Discard any drugs which have expired.

11. Introduce pill organizers for elderly patients. A pill organizer for the weekly supply of medications can prevent omitting or duplicating medications. Twenty-three percent of nursing home admissions are related to patient's inability to take medications correctly.

12. Provide a written chart to the patient who is taking several medications per day. A study entitled "Improving Memory Function in Elderly Adults with Contextual Cues" by Dr. Denise C. Park, University of Georgia-Gerontology Center, Athens, Georgia found the following:

A seven-day medication organizer with compartments for different times of the day was correctly loaded with their medications. We followed these patients for several weeks, measuring adherence errors using special microelectronic recording devices to detect exactly what time and date the medication was taken. Some patients in these studies also received computer-generated organizational charts to help them organize and remember to take their medications. The major findings from these studies were (a) the oldest-old (people over age 75) made significantly more adherence errors than people aged 60-74; (b) the organizers alone showed some evidence of enhancing adherence, but the strongest effects occurred when combined with an organizational chart.

SAMPLE CHART

| medication frequency instructions | date Sun 5/15 | date Mon 5/16 | date Tues 5/17 | date Wed 5/18 | date Thurs 5/19 | date Fri 5/20 | date Sat 5/21 |
|---|---|---|---|---|---|---|---|
| Synthroid 150 mcg once a day every morning Thyroid | 8 AM | 8 AM | 8 AM | 8 AM | 8 AM | 8 AM | 8 AM |
| Coumadin 5 mg po Mon Wed Fri anticoagulant watch for bleeding | | 8 AM | | 8 AM | | 8 AM | |
| Coumadin 2.5 mg Sun Tues Thurs Sat Anticoagulant | 8 AM | | 8 AM | | 8 AM | | 8 AM |
| Digoxin 0.125 mg qd po Heart medication call MD if HR<60 | 8 AM | 8 AM | 8 AM | 8 AM | 8 AM | 8 AM | 8 AM |
| Lasix 10 mg qAM po water pill (diuretic) | 8 AM | 8 AM | 8 AM | 8 AM | 8 AM | 8 AM | 8 AM |
| K-lyte 20 mEq in 8 ounces of juice with meals three time a day Potassium supplement | 8 AM 12 N 5 PM | 8 AM 12 N 5 PM | 8 AM 12 N 5 PM | 8 AM 12 N 5 PM | 8 AM 12 N 5 PM | 8 AM 12 N 5 PM | 8 AM 12 N 5 PM |

Develop your own chart for the patient using the above as a sample.

## Patient Teaching

A California homecare infusion agency has a patient with a PICC catheter (brand name for a catheter inserted in an antecubital vein with the tip positioned in the superior vena cava), that has been patent and infection free for 2 years. This demonstrates that it is possible for the care givers to give excellent safe care after outstanding patient teaching on the part of the home health nurse.

## Methods for Patient Teaching

1. Identify what the patient really needs to know to perform the procedure safely, not what would be nice for him/her to know.

2. Only instruct 3-4 points per session. In your teaching keep it short, specific, and simple. The average adult can remember only 5-7 points at a time. A written step by step list may be helpful to guide the caregiver in the procedure. Avoid medical terminology that may not be understood.

3. Reinforce the care givers learning by compliments, smiles, and a nod of the head for getting it right. Let the family know that you are there to encourage, support and teach.

4. Incorporate your teaching into everyday patient care. Talk to your patient, as you are doing a procedure or giving a medication, about the purpose of each step or each medication. Hearing it over and over again helps to reinforce learning.

5. Have the care giver do a return demonstration after having observed you do the procedure. If the procedure is complicated, it may require several return demonstrations before the sequence of steps is mastered correctly.

## Drug Calculations with Homecare Patients

The following are some examples of drug calculation problems that the nurse may encounter in the home.

1. Dressing changes with solutions to clean and promote wound healing. It may be a postoperative wound that has not healed completely or a diabetic with cellulitis of the leg.

2. Dosing of the elderly based on weight and creatinine clearance.

3. Antibiotic administration with a midline intravenous catheter. Measurement of Peak and Trough levels of the serum concentration of the antibiotic.

## Solutions for External Use

A stock solution is a mixture of a pure drug dissolved in a solution. Some examples of stock solutions are Betadine 10% and Hydrogen Peroxide 3%. These are prepared commercially and can be purchased at any pharmacy. Dakins 2.5 % is prepared by the pharmacist under a laminar flow hood. Stock solutions are not prepared in the home. Preparation requires an accurate metric scale, sterile diluent, and sterile containers. The nurse may prepare a weaker solution from a stock solution. The formula method provides a safe way to solve these problems with numerous variables. The ratio proportion method may also be used, but sometimes it is safer to only put the numbers into a formula.

# Using the Formula Method: Solution Dilutions

■ Problem: Prepare 250 mL of a 1.5% solution (half strength solution 3% x ½ = 1.5%) of hydrogen peroxide from a stock solution of 3% hydrogen peroxide. Use normal saline as a diluent. Irrigate the wound with half strength peroxide solution.

---

V1C1=V2C2 DILUENT = V1-V2

To solve for $V1 = \dfrac{V2 \times C2}{C1}$    V1 = Final volume you want to prepare.

To solve for $V2 = \dfrac{V1 \times C1}{C2}$    V2 = Volume of stock solution you will need for dilution.

To solve for $C1 = \dfrac{V2 \times C2}{V1}$    C1 = Concentration of the solution you wish to prepare.

To solve for $C2 = \dfrac{V1 \times C1}{V2}$    C2 = Concentration of the stock solution you will use.

---

A.  V1— Final volume you want to prepare?

Answer: 250 mL

B.  C1 —Concentration of the solution you wish to prepare?

Answer: 1.5% solution of peroxide

C.  V2— Volume of stock solution you will need for dilution?

Answer: unknown

D.  C2— Concentration of the stock solution you will use?

Answer: 3% hydrogen peroxide

E.  What is the unknown and the formula needed?

Answer: V2 = V1xC1/C2

F.  How much stock solution is needed?

$$V2 = \frac{250 \text{ mL x } 1.5\%}{3\%} = 125 \text{ mL}$$

Answer: 125 mL of hydrogen peroxide

G.  How much diluent (normal saline) is needed? (V1-V2) 250 mL - 125 mL = 125 mL

Answer : 125 mL of normal saline

■ In summary, to prepare 250 mL of a 1.5% solution of hydrogen peroxide from a 3% stock solution 125 mL of stock solution and 125 mL diluent—normal saline. Half strength solutions are one part stock solution to one part diluent. Supplies needed: sterile irrigation set for measurement, 3% hydrogen peroxide, plus a 500 mL bottle of normal saline for irrigation.

1. The physician orders (2.5%) or ¼ strength solution of Betadine for a foot soak for your home care patient. Prepare 800 mL of (2.5%) ¼ strength Betadine. The stock solution is Betadine 10%. The diluent is normal saline. How much Betadine do you need and how much normal saline do you need?

    A. V1— Final volume you want to prepare?  _____

    B. C1 — Concentration of the solution you wish to prepare?  _____

    C. V2— Volume of stock solution you will need for dilution?  _____

    D. C2— Concentration of the stock solution you will use?  _____

    E. What is the unknown and what is the formula?  _____

    F. How much stock solution is needed?  _____

    G. How much diluent is needed? (V1-V2)  _____

2. You have only 75 mL of Betadine 10% stock solution left in the bottle. You wish to prepare a ¼ or 2.5% strength solution from the 75 mL of Betadine using normal saline as the diluent.

    A. V1— Final volume you want to prepare?  _____

    B. C1 — Concentration of the solution you wish to prepare?  _____

    C. V2— Volume of stock solution you will need for dilution?  _____

    D. C2— Concentration of the stock solution you will use?  _____

    E. What is the unknown and what is the formula?  _____

    F. What is the final volume needed to make a 2.5% solution from 75 mL of Betadine?_____

    G. How much diluent is needed? (V1-V2)  _____

**Note:** *Quarter strength solutions are 1 part stock solution to three parts diluent.*

3. You wish to prepare 500 mL of a 0.1% solution for a vinegar douche. Stock solution of vinegar is 5% acidity. Diluent is tap water.

    A. V1— Final volume you want to prepare?  _____

    B. C1 — Concentration of the solution you wish to prepare?  _____

    C. V2— Volume of stock solution you will need for dilution?  _____

    D. C2— Concentration of the stock solution you will use?  _____

    E. What is the unknown and what is the formula?  _____

    F. How much stock solution is needed?  _____

    G. How much diluent is needed? (V1-V2)  _____

V1C1=V2C2 DILUENT = V1-V2

To solve for V1 = $\frac{V2 \times C2}{C1}$     V1 = Final volume you want to prepare.

To solve for V2 = $\frac{V1 \times C1}{C2}$     V2 = Volume of stock solution you will need for dilution.

To solve for C1 = $\frac{V2 \times C2}{V1}$     C1 = Concentration of the solution you wish to prepare.

To solve for C2 = $\frac{V1 \times C1}{V2}$     C2 = Concentration of the stock solution you will use.

4. Prepare 60 mL of (1.5%) or a half strength solution of hydrogen peroxide from a 3% stock solution of hydrogen peroxide for a mouthwash. The patient has had oral surgery. Use normal saline as the diluent.

   A. V1— Final volume you want to prepare?                    _____

   B. C1 — Concentration of the solution you wish to prepare?     _____

   C. V2— Volume of stock solution you will need for dilution is?_____

   D. C2— Concentration of the stock solution you will use?     _____

   E. What is the unknown and what is the formula?             _____

   F. How much stock solution is needed?                       _____

   G. How much diluent is needed? (V1-V2)                      _____

**Note:** *Half strength solutions are one part stock solution to one part diluent.*

Answers: Chapter 12, Solutions
1. A. 800 B. 2.5% C. unknown D. 10% E. V2 = V1x C1 / C2 F. 200 mL of Betadine G. 600 mL normal saline.
2 . A. unknown B. 2.5 % C. 75 mL D. 10% E. V1 = V2xC2 / C1 F. 300 mL G. 225mL normal saline.
3. A. 500 mL B. 0.1% C. unknown D. 5% E. V2 = V1xC1/C2 F. 10 mL of vinegar G. 490 mL of tap water.
4. A. 60 mL B. 1.5 C. unknown D. 3% E. V2 = V1XC1/C2 F. 30 mL hydrogen peroxide. G. 30 mL of normal saline.

# ELDERLY DRUG DOSAGE BASED ON BODY WEIGHT AND/OR CREATININE CLEARANCE

Decline in two major organs, the kidney and liver, have the most profound effect on drug distribution, metabolism and excretion. Renal function may decline by 50% between the ages of 50 and 90. Liver size and blood flow may decrease as much as 40% between 40 and 80 years of age. This functional decline can lead to drug accumulation because the liver may not be able to break the drug down and the kidneys may not be able to eliminate the drug as readily.

The functional decline of organ systems with aging makes the safe range for drug dosage in the elderly different than young and middle-aged adults. It is recommended that nurses working with the elderly refer to a drug handbook that addresses the needs of the elderly. The American Pharmaceutical Association recommends *Geriatric Dosage Handbook* by Todd Semla, Judith Belzer and Martin Higbee.

The physician has ordered Valium (diazepam) 5 mg HS prn for anxiety. The patient is 70 years of age and has night time anxiety. In the *Geriatric Dosage Handbook* under Geriatric Considerations it states "due to its long-acting metabolite, Valium (diazepam) is not considered a drug of choice in the elderly . . . long acting benzodiaxepines have been associated with falls in the elderly. . . . The Health Care Financing Administration discourages the use of this agent in long-term care facilities. Under Pharmacokinetics it states the half life is 20-50 hours and in the elderly the half life may increase to 90 hours."

*Definition of half-life is the length of time required to reduce a drug's original plasma concentration by 50%, which is determined by bio-transformation and excretion and does not vary with drug dosage.* A 5 mg dose of Valium with a half life of 50 hours is 2.5 mg at one half life and 1.25 mg at 2 half lives or 100 hours. So it is obvious that if the Valium is given every night, it will have an accumulative effect over time, especially with the elderly where the half life may be up to 90 hours.

Is Valium 5 mg HS prn for a 70 year old patient safe? Answer: No
The nurse should notify the physician that Valium is not recommended for the elderly and the pharmacist recommends Ativan (lorazepam) as a better choice due to its short half life of 10-16 hours.

If an elderly patient has been taking Valium, the nurse should be especially alert to signs and symptoms of an adverse drug reaction. For example, a 70 year old male became confused at night and his coordination suddenly deteriorated as evidenced by his spilling the urinal. In reviewing the medication history, the nurse observed that the patient had been given Valium at bedtime. It was discontinued by the physician and the confusion and lack of coordination disappeared.

All patients should be observed for adverse drug reactions, but the nurse must be especially vigilant when assessing the elderly. Never assume that a change in behavior is because the patient is elderly.

Serum creatinine and creatinine clearance are different ways to determine renal function. So they are useful tools for adjusting drug dosages in the elderly where some renal impairment may exist. According to Jeff Punch, M.D., of the University of Michigan Division of Transplantation, "Creatinine is a protein produced by the muscle and released into the blood. . . . The creatinine level in the serum is determined by the rate it is being removed, which is roughly a measure of kidney function. The serum creatinine is determined by drawing a blood sample and the normal range for an adult is **0.7-1.5 mg/dl**. Creatinine clearance is technically the amount of blood that is cleared of creatinine by the kidneys per time period. It is expressed in mL per min."

Creatinine clearance is determined by obtaining a 24 hour urine sample. Normal creatinine clearance is **70-130 mL/min**.

Ranges used as a measure of renal impairment are:

Normal > 100 mL/min

Mild renal impairment 40-60 mL/min

Moderate renal impairment 10-40 mL/min

Severe renal impairment that may require dialysis <10 mL/min

*Practice Problems*

# DRUG DOSAGE BASED ON ACTUAL CREATININE CLEARANCE

1. Ms. Rightmyer, an 85 year old nursing home resident, is suffering from frequent urination with a burning sensation. A urine sample is sent for culture and sensitivity. Her creatinine clearance is 18 mL/minute.

▪ *The physician orders Zinacef (cefuroxime) 1.5 g IV piggyback q 8 h.*

The *Geriatric Dosage Handbook* by Semla, Beizer and Higbee states dosing interval in renal impairment is:

creatinine clearance > 20 mL/min Administer 750 mg to 1500 mg q 8 h.
creatinine clearance 10-20 mL/min administer 750 mg q 12 hours
creatinine clearance <10 mL/min administer 750 mg q 24 hours

Is Zinacef 1.5 g IV q8h safe for this patient? _____

2. Mr. Stokley, a home care patient, has been diagnosed with beta hemolytic streptococcus.

▪ *The physician orders Keflex 500 mg po q 12 h. Mr Stokley's creatinine clearance is 30 mL/min.*

The *Geriatric Dosage Handbook* by Semla, Beizer and Higbee states dosing interval in renal impairment is oral 250-1000 mg po.

creatinine clearance 10-40 mL/min administer every 8 to 12 hours
creatinine clearance 15-10 mL/min administer every 12 hours
creatinine clearance <5 mL/min administer 12-24 hours

Is Keflex 500 mg po q 12 h safe for this patient? _____

Answers: Chapter 12, 1-2, Actual Creatinine Clearance
1. No, the dosage for Ms. Rightmyer should be reduced to 750 mg q 12 hours.
2. Yes, the dosage interval for a patient with a creatinine clearance of 30 mL/min is every 8-12 hours.

# FORMULAS FOR ESTIMATING CREATININE CLEARANCE

Serum creatinine levels are more easily obtained since it involves only a blood sample versus a 24 hour urine collection. The Cockroft-Gault formula to determine estimates of creatinine clearance is as follows.

Crockroft-Gault Formula—Males

$$\frac{[\,(140 - age\,) \times weight\ in\ kg\,]}{72 \times serum\ creatinine} = creatinine\ clearance$$

Crockroft-Gault Formula—Females

$$\frac{[\,(140 - age\,) \times weight\ in\ kg\,]}{72 \times serum\ creatinine} = creatinine\ clearance \times 0.85$$

Formulas for Adjusted Weight for Patients who are not their ideal body weight.

current weight in kg - ideal weight in kg = _____ x 0.4 = _____ + ideal wt = _____ adjusted weight

# Male Patient Using the Cockroft-Gault Formula

■ Mr. Castle is a 48 year old male patient weighing 207 pounds or 94 kilograms. He has sustained multiple rib fractures. He is presently a home care patient who acquired pneumonia with pseudomonas aeruginosa as the cultured organism. His serum creatinine is 1.8 mg/dl. What is the creatinine clearance?

$$\frac{[\,(140 - 48\,)\; x\; 94\; kg\,]}{72\; x\; serum\; creatinine\; 1.8} = \frac{8648}{129.6} = 66.7\; mL/min\; creatinine\; clearance$$

Answer: The estimated creatinine clearance is 66.7

■ *The physician orders Penicillin G 5 million units IV PB q 6 h. Mr. Stokley's estimated creatinine is 67 mL/min.*

The drug handbook states that: For a creatinine clearance of > 30 mL/min administer Penicillin 3-5 million units every 6 hours. For a creatinine clearance of 10-30 mL/min administer Penicillin G 3-5 million units every 8-12 h For a creatinine clearance of < 10 administer Penicillin G 3-5 million units every 12-18 hours.

Is this dosage safe for an estimated creatinine clearance of 67mL/min?

Answer: Yes the every six hour dosage interval is safe for patients with a creatinine clearance of greater than 30 mL/min

# Female Patient Using the Cockroft-Gault Formula

■ Ms. Lindberg is a 65 year old female patient, who is 11 days status post ruptured appendix and appendectomy. Her serum creatinine is 0.6 mg/dl. She weighs 68 kg which is her ideal body weight. What is her estimated creatinine clearance?

$$\frac{[\,(140 - 65)\; x\; 68\,]}{72\; x\; 0.6} = \frac{5100}{43} = 118.6\; x\; 0.85 = 100.8\; estimated\; creatinine\; clearance$$

# For Patients who are not their ideal body weight

■ Mr. James is very overweight. Adjust the weight for an obese patient for the Cockroft-Gault formula. Mr James, who is 60 years has an ideal weight of 85 kg. His current weight is 126 kg. His serum creatinine is 1.7 mg/dl

current weight in kg - ideal weight in kg = _____ x 0.4 = _____ + ideal wt = _____adjusted weight

126 -85 = 41 x 0.4 = 16.4   16.4 + 85 = 101 kg

Answer: Use 101 kg as the adjusted weight of the obese patient in the Cockroft-Gault formula.

$$\frac{[\,(140 - 60\,)\; x\; 101\,]}{72\; x\; 1.7} = \frac{8080}{122.4} = 66\; estimated\; creatinine\; clearance$$

1. Mr. Blackman is a 60 year old male who weighs 75 kg. This is close to his ideal body weight. His serum creatinine is 1 mg/dl. Using The Cockroft-Gault formula calculate the estimated creatinine clearance.

2. Mr. Miller is a 74 year old male patient who weighs 89 kg. This is his ideal body weight. His serum creatinine is 1.7 mg/dl. Using The Cockroft-Gault formula calculate the estimated creatinine clearance.

3. Ms. Rust is a 50 year old female who weighs 62 kg. This is her ideal body weight. Her serum creatinine is 0.7 mg/dl. Using The Cockroft-Gault formula for female patients calculate the estimated creatinine clearance.

4. Ms. Bado is an 85 year old female who weighs 55 kg. This is her ideal body weight. Her serum creatinine is 1.2 mg/dl. Using The Cockroft-Gault formula for female patients, calculate the estimated creatinine clearance.

5. Mr. Hines is 65 years old and weighs 110 kg. However his ideal body weight is 80 kg. Calculate the dose adjusted weight.

6. Mr. Hines is a 65 year old obese male. His dose adjusted weight is 92 kg. His serum creatinine is 1.3 mg/dl. Using The Cockroft-Gault formula for male patients, calculate the estimated creatinine clearance.

Answers: Chapter 12, 1-6 estimated creatinine clearance.
1. The estimated creatinine clearance is 83 mL/minute
2. The estimated clearance is 48 mL/minute
3. The estimated creatinine clearance is 94 mL/minute
4. The estimated creatinine clearance is 30 mL/minute
5. The adjusted weight is 92 kg.
6. The estimated creatinine clearance is 73.7 mL/minute.

# Therapeutic Drug Monitoring

Home care patients may be sent home on drugs that have a narrow therapeutic range which requires therapeutic drug monitoring. The following problems relate to therapeutic drug monitoring. The therapeutic range is the amount of the drug in the blood serum that will produce the desired effect without producing toxicity. The following problems will require a variety of drug calculation skills which you have previously encountered.

1.   Mr. Watsabaugh has a post operative wound infection which cultured the organism Klebsiella. He weighs 190 lbs or 86 kg. The physician orders gentamicin 50 mg IV PB q 8 h. Mr. Watsabaugh is started on the gentamicin in the hospital and was then discharged home to continue IV therapy with home health care nursing. The drug handbook states that the IV dose of gentamicin is 1.5-2 mg per kg divided in three doses.
   Is gentamicin 50 mg IV PB q 8 h safe? _____

2.   The pharmacy has delivered a 24 hour supply of gentamicin 50 mg in 50 mL of D5W to Mr. Watsabaugh's home. The home health nurse draws the trough level of gentamicin at 1330 which is 30 minutes before the 1400 gentamicin is due. A peak level of gentamicin (serum specimen) is ordered following the 2 P.M. (1400) dose of gentamicin. There is an IV pump to deliver the gentamicin. To get an accurate peak level the gentamicin must be given over exactly 30 minutes and a peak level drawn 30 minutes following the infusion.
   What is the correct IV infusion rate? _____

3.   Mr. Watsabaugh's peak gentamicin level is 8 mcg/mL and his trough level is 0.95 mcg/ mL.

**Note:** *The* Geriatric Dosage Handbook *states the therapeutic peak level is 4-8 mcg/mL and the therapeutic trough level is <2mcg/mL. The MIC (minimum inhibitory concentration) reported from the lab indicates 0.5 mcg/mL is sufficient to inhibit bacterial growth.*

   A. Does Mr. Watsabaugh's peak level fall within the therapeutic range? _____
   B. Does the trough level fall within the therapeutic range?         _____
   C. Does the trough level fall above the MIC?                        _____

4. Ms. Peterson, a 72 year old patient, is on a maintenance dose of digoxin 0.125 mg qd. She walks ½ mile 3 times per week. A digoxin blood level was obtained 8 hours after she last took her morning digoxin.

**Note:** *The normal therapeutic range for digoxin is 0.5-2 ng/mL.*

The home health nurse reviews the lab report for the digoxin level and finds Mrs. Peterson's level to be 0.4 ng/mL.

Is the maintenance dose of digoxin 0.125 mg qd maintaining the digoxin level within the therapeutic range?

_____

Answers: Chapter 12, 1-4, Therapeutic Range
1. Yes the safe range for a patient weighing 86 kg is 43-57 mg q 8 h.
2. Set the infusion pump at 100 mL per hour to deliver 50 mL over 30 minutes.
3. A. Yes B. Yes C. Yes
4. No it falls below the therapeutic range. Exercise in elderly will reduce serum concentrations of digoxin due to increased skeletal uptake.

# 13

## Chapter Thirteen

## Dimensional Analysis

Co-author: Bonnie C. Benson, MS, RN
Professor of Nursing
Westminster College, St. Mark's-
Westminster School of Nursing
Salt Lake City, Utah

# Dimensional Analysis

Drug calculations may be done by three methods: (1) ratio proportion, (2) formula and (3) dimensional analysis. The third method of drug calculations, dimensional analysis, will be the focus of this chapter. It may be helpful to compare the first two methods, utilized in the previous chapters 1-5, 7 and 9. The formula method was shown primarily with sample problems involving infusion rates, found in chapters 7 (p.130), 8 and 11. Additionally, for purposes of comparison and contrast, the formula method was situated next to the ratio proportion method in chapter 2 (pp.48-49) and chapter 9 (pp. 174-175). Finally, formulas have been summarized on pocket guides at the end of this book.

## Dimensional Analysis—A Problem Solving Method

Dimensional analysis is a problem-solving method or process whereby an individual converts a given unit of measurement (a dimension involving weight, volume or length) to another unit of measurement desired as an answer to the problem. Some of you may already be familiar with this method, as it is often used in chemistry and physics courses. It also may be referred to as the unit factor or label factor method. The problem is set up so that the starting factor is multiplied by the conversion factor(s) expressed in fraction format, so that unwanted factors are canceled and only the label factor (answer) remains.

## Advantages of Dimensional Analysis

1. It may be used for almost all types of dosage calculation problems, thus eliminating or minimizing the need for formulas.

2. It may be used for both simple and complex problems because multiple conversions can be set up in one single problem.

3. It enables an individual to critically analyze what type of answer is needed and to select needed information and appropriate conversions for the calculation.

4. It reduces confusion regarding whether to divide or multiply, and it may simplify the math calculation through cancellation or reduction of numbers in the fraction(s).

## Steps to Dimensional Analysis

(Shown in sample problems on pages 228-234 and 236)
1. Identify the starting factor and the label factor.
The starting factor is the given unit of measurement (dimension), commonly the prescribed quantity or rate (the physicians order). The label factor is the desired unit of measurement in your answer, usually the dimension that must be measured to give the medicine or fluid to the patient.

2. Determine the appropriate conversion(s).
Two types of conversion factors may be used: (1) memorized conversions whereby one system or unit of measurement is converted to another such as 1 gr = 60 mg and (2) equivalents printed on the drug label such as 1 tablet = 50 mg or on the intravenous tubing box 1 mL = 10 gtts. The conversion factor is expressed as a fraction in which the numerator is equal to the denominator. The position of numerator and denominator may be reversed in any conversion because of their equality (1:1 or 1/1 proportion; or 1 gr/60mg or 60 mg / 1 gr).

3. Arrange the problem so that each label (unit of measurement) not wanted in the answer can be canceled by its placement as a numerator and a consecutive denominator. Generally, the starting factor and the label factor (answer) should be placed as numerators in the problem setup.

4. Cancel unwanted labels (units of measurement) and circle all remaining label factors or the units in your answer. Cross out matching units of measurement, but do not cross out the numbers next to each numerator and consecutive denominator.

5. Reduce numbers to lowest terms.
Divide a number in the numerator and a number in the denominator by the same number, thus not changing the ultimate value.

6. Multiply across the numerators. Multiply across the denominators. Divide the total numerator by the total denominator, creating a whole number or a number with a decimal point as your answer. This is simple math. The need for a rounded or precise answer will vary according to the type of problem.

7. Determine if the answer is reasonable such as a realistic volume for an injection, or a reasonable number of tablets, or the number of kilograms is less than the number of the pounds. Double check the calculations if the answer does not seem reasonable. Check the conversion factors. Double check the placement and cancellation of units of measurement. All dimensions should be eliminated other than the label factor(s) (answer). The label factor(s) should be in the same position on both sides of the equation (usually as a numerator). Double check the math with a calculator. If the numbers were reduced in step 5, double check the math using the original numbers. If a common fraction in the numerator or denominator makes it confusing, change it to a decimal.

In the remaining pages of this chapter, sample problems using dimensional analysis will be provided. The same or similar sample problems were done by the ratio proportion or formula methods in previous chapters. Page references will be provided for practice problems to calculate by the dimensional analysis method.

# Method: Dimensional Analysis
# Units of Measure

■ *How many feet are in 24 inches?*

1. Identify the starting factor and the label factor.
Starting factor 24 inches          Label factor (answer) _____ feet

2. Determine the appropriate conversion: 1 foot = 12 inches (memorized).

$$\frac{1 \text{ foot}}{12 \text{ inches}} \text{ or } \frac{12 \text{ inches}}{1 \text{ foot}}$$

3. Arrange the problem so that each label (unit of measurement) not wanted in the answer can be canceled by its placement as a numerator and a consecutive denominator.

$$\frac{24 \text{ inches}}{1} \text{ X } \frac{1 \text{ foot}}{12 \text{ inches}} = \underline{\hspace{1cm}} \text{ feet}$$

4. Cancel unwanted labels (units of measurement) and circle all remaining label factors (answer).

$$\frac{24 \text{ in} \cancel{\text{ches}}}{1} \text{ X } \frac{1 \boxed{\text{foot}}}{12 \text{ in} \cancel{\text{ches}}} = \underline{\hspace{1cm}} \text{ feet}$$

5. Reduce numbers to lowest terms.

$$\frac{\overset{2}{\cancel{24}}}{1} \text{ X } \frac{1 \boxed{\text{foot}}}{\underset{1}{\cancel{12}}} = \underline{\hspace{1cm}} \text{ feet}$$

6. Multiply across the numerators. Multiply across the denominators. Divide the total numerator by the total denominator, creating a whole number or a number with a decimal point as your answer.

$$\frac{2}{1} \text{ X } \frac{1 \boxed{\text{foot}}}{1} = 2 \text{ feet}$$

■ **In summary, 24 inches equals 2 feet.**

# Method: Dimensional Analysis
# Oral Tablets or Capsules

*The physician orders Lanoxin (digoxin) 0.25 mg po qd.*

1. Identify the starting factor and the label factor.

Starting factor (order) 0.25 mg          Label factor (answer) _____ tab (tablets)

2. Determine the appropriate conversion: 0.125 mg = 1 tab (drug label).

$$\frac{0.125 \text{ mg}}{1 \text{ tab}} \quad \text{or} \quad \frac{1 \text{ tab}}{0.125 \text{ mg}}$$

3. Arrange the problem so that each label (unit of measurement) not wanted in the answer can be canceled by its placement as a numerator and a consecutive denominator.

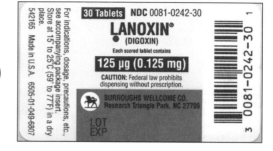

$$\frac{0.25 \text{ mg}}{1} \times \frac{1 \text{ tab}}{0.125 \text{ mg}} = \underline{\hspace{1cm}} \text{ tab}$$

4. Cancel unwanted labels (units of measurement) and circle all remaining label factors (answer).

$$\frac{0.25 \cancel{\text{mg}}}{1} \times \frac{1 \, \boxed{\text{tab}}}{0.125 \cancel{\text{mg}}} = \underline{\hspace{1cm}} \text{ tab}$$

5. Reduce numbers to lowest terms.

$$\frac{\overset{2}{\cancel{0.25}}}{1} \times \frac{1 \, \boxed{\text{tab}}}{\underset{1}{\cancel{0.125}}} = \underline{\hspace{1cm}} \text{ tab}$$

6. Multiply across the numerators. Multiply across the denominators. Divide the total numerators by the total denominators, creating a whole number or a number with a decimal point as your answer.

$$\frac{2}{1} \times \frac{1 \, \boxed{\text{tab}}}{1} = 2 \text{ tab}$$

**In summary, to give Lanoxin 0.25 mg to the patient, give 2 tablets. Two tablets = 0.25 mg.**

Note: *Look at the answer and ask, is this answer reasonable. If it is not, check the numbers and recalculate. Do problems 1-25 starting on page 51 in chapter 2. Use the back cover to look up conversion factors if not yet memorized.*

# Method: Dimensional Analysis
# Oral Liquids

*The physician orders Claritin (loratadine) 3 mg po qd.*

1. Identify the starting factor and the label factor.
Starting factor (order) 3 mg. Label factor (answer) _____ mL

2. Determine the appropriate conversions: 10 mg = 10 mL (drug label)

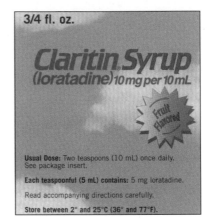

$$\text{drug label}$$

$$\frac{10 \text{ mg}}{10 \text{ mL}} \text{ or } \frac{10 \text{ mL}}{10 \text{ mg}}$$

3. Arrange the problem so that each label (unit of measurement) not wanted in the answer can be canceled by its placement as a numerator and a consecutive denominator.

$$\frac{3 \text{ mg}}{1} \text{ X } \frac{10 \text{ mL}}{10 \text{ mg}} = \text{_____ mL}$$

4. Cancel unwanted labels (units of measurement) and circle all remaining label factors (answer).

$$\frac{3 \text{ m\!\!\!/g}}{1} \text{ X } \frac{10 \text{ (mL)}}{10 \text{ m\!\!\!/g}} = \text{_____ mL}$$

5. Multiply across the numerators. Multiply across the denominators. Divide the total numerators by the total denominators, creating a whole number or a number with a decimal point as your answer.

$$\frac{3}{1} \text{ X } \frac{1}{1} = 3 \text{ mL}$$

**In summary, to give Claritin 3 mg to the patient, 3 mL should be given.**

**Note:** *Look at the answer and ask is this answer reasonable. If it is not, check the numbers and recalculate.*
   *Do problems 1-25 starting on page 51 in chapter 2. Use the back cover to look up conversion factors if not yet memorized.*

# Method: Dimensional Analysis
# Injectable Drugs

*The physician orders Demerol 35 mg IM now.*

1. Identify the starting factor and the label factor.
Starting factor (order) 35 mg            Label factor (answer) _____ mL

2. Determine the appropriate conversion. Obtain this from the medication label. No memorized conversions are needed in this problem. The units are the same for both desired dose and dosage on hand: 100 mg = 1 mL

$$\frac{100 \text{ mg}}{1 \text{ mL}} \text{ or } \frac{1 \text{ mg}}{100 \text{ mg}}$$

3. Arrange the problem so that each label (unit of measurement) not wanted in the answer can be canceled by its placement as a numerator and a consecutive denominator.

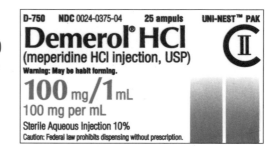

$$\frac{35 \text{ mg}}{1} \text{ X } \frac{1 \text{ mL}}{100 \text{ mg}} = \underline{\hspace{1cm}} \text{ mL}$$

4. Cancel unwanted labels (units of measurement) and circle all remaining label factors (answer).

$$\frac{35 \text{ m\cancel{g}}}{1} \text{ X } \frac{1\,\widehat{\text{mL}}}{100 \text{ m\cancel{g}}} = \underline{\hspace{1cm}} \text{ mL}$$

5. Multiply across the numerators. Multiply across the denominators. Divide the total numerators by the total denominators, creating a whole number or a number with a decimal point as your answer.

$$\frac{35}{1} \text{ X } \frac{1\,\widehat{\text{mL}}}{100} = \frac{35}{100} = 0.35 \text{ mL}$$

**In summary, to give Demerol 35 mg to the patient, give 0.35 mL.**

Note: *Look at the answer and ask is this answer reasonable. If it is not, check the numbers and recalculate.*
   *Do practice problems 26-55 starting on page 63 in Chapter 2.*

# Method: Dimensional Analysis
# Injectable Drugs

*The physician orders ampicillin 0.25 g IM.*

1. Identify the starting factor and the label factor.
Starting factor (order) 0.25 g           Label factor (answer) _____ mL

2. Determine the appropriate conversions. 250 mg = 1 mL (Drug label) 1 g = 1000 mg (memorized conversion).

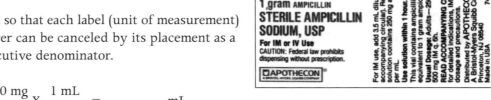

Memorized conversion

$$\frac{1 g}{1000 mg} \text{ or } \frac{1000 mg}{1 g} \quad \text{and} \quad \frac{250 mg}{1 mL} \text{ or } \frac{1 mL}{250 mg}$$

Drug label

NDC 0015-7404-20
NSN 6505-00-993-3518
EQUIVALENT TO

**1 gram** AMPICILLIN

**STERILE AMPICILLIN**
**SODIUM, USP**

**For IM or IV Use**
CAUTION: Federal law prohibits
dispensing without prescription.

◻APOTHECON®
A BRISTOL-MYERS SQUIBB COMPANY

3. Arrange the problem so that each label (unit of measurement) not wanted in the answer can be canceled by its placement as a numerator and a consecutive denominator.

$$\frac{0.25 g}{1} \text{ X } \frac{1000 mg}{1 g} \text{ X } \frac{1 mL}{250 mg} = \text{_____ mL}$$

4. Cancel unwanted labels (units of measurement) and circle all remaining label factors (answer).

$$\frac{0.25 \cancel{g}}{1} \text{ X } \frac{1000 \cancel{mg}}{1 \cancel{g}} \text{ X } \frac{1 \boxed{mL}}{250 \cancel{mg}} = \text{_____ mL}$$

5. Reduce numbers to lowest terms.

$$\frac{0.25}{1} \text{ X } \frac{\overset{4}{\cancel{1000}}}{1} \text{ X } \frac{1 \boxed{mL}}{\underset{1}{\cancel{250}}} = \text{_____ mL}$$

6. Multiply across the numerators. Multiply across the denominators. Divide the total numerators by the total denominators, creating a whole number or a number with a decimal point as your answer.

$$\frac{0.25}{1} \text{ X } \frac{4}{1} \text{ X } \frac{1 mL}{1} = 0.25 \text{ X } 4 = 1 mL$$

**In summary, to give ampicillin 0.25 g, give 1 mL.**

**Note:** *Look at the answer and ask is this answer reasonable. If it is not, check the numbers and recalculate.*
*Do problems 1-30, starting on page 91 in Chapter 5.*

# Method: Dimensional Analysis
# Calculation of a Drug Dosage
# which Requires a Memorized Conversion

■ *A physician ordered morphine sulfate gr 1/8 IM q4h prn for pain. Morphine sulfate 15 mg is available from pharmacy.*

1. Identify starting factor and label factor.
 Starting factor (order) gr $\frac{1}{8}$. Label factor (answer) _____ mL

2. Identify the appropriate conversions.

| Memorized conversion | | | Drug label | | |
|---|---|---|---|---|---|
| 1 gr = 60 mg or | $\frac{1 \text{ gr}}{60 \text{ mg}}$ or | $\frac{60 \text{ mg}}{1 \text{ gr}}$ | 15 mg = 1 mL or | $\frac{15 \text{ mg}}{1 \text{ mL}}$ or | $\frac{1 \text{mL}}{15 \text{ mg}}$ |

3. Arrange the problem so that each label (unit of measurement) not wanted in the answer can be canceled by its placement as a numerator and a consecutive denominator.

order memorized conversion drug label

$$\frac{\text{gr } 1}{8} \; X \; \frac{60 \text{ mg}}{\text{gr } 1} \; X \; \frac{1 \text{ mL}}{15 \text{ mg}} = \text{_____ mL}$$

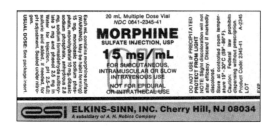

4. Cancel unwanted labels (units of measurement) and circle all remaining label factors (answer).

$$\frac{\cancel{\text{gr}} \text{ 1}}{8} \; X \; \frac{60 \cancel{\text{ mg}}}{\cancel{\text{gr}} \text{ 1}} \; X \; \frac{1 \;\textcircled{mL}}{15 \cancel{\text{ mg}}} = \text{_____ mL}$$

5. Reduce numbers to lowest terms. Convert the fraction to a decimal.

$$\frac{1}{8} \; X \; \frac{\overset{4}{\cancel{60}}}{1} \; X \; \frac{1 \;\textcircled{mL}}{\underset{1}{\cancel{15}}} = \text{_____ mL}$$

6. Multiply across the numerators. Multiply across the denominators. Divide the total numerators by the total denominators, creating a whole number or a number with a decimal point as the answer.

$$\frac{1}{8} \; X \; \frac{4}{1} \; X \; \frac{1 \;\textcircled{mL}}{1} = \frac{4}{8} = 0.5 \text{ mL}$$

■ **In summary, gr 1/8 = 0.5 mL. Give 0.5 mL.**

**Note:** *Look at the answer, and ask is this answer reasonable? If it is not check the numbers and recalculate. In this problem the dose on hand and the physician's order are not in the same units. The problem required a memorized conversion.*

*Do problems 1-30 starting on page 91 chapter 5. Use the back cover to look up conversion factors if not yet memorized. Also do problems 1-46, starting on page 85 in Chapter 4 to practice conversions.*

# Method: Dimensional Analysis
# Pediatric Conversion of Pounds and Ounces to Kilograms

■ *An infant's weight is 11 lbs 4 oz.*

## A. How many kilograms does this infant weigh?

1. Starting factor: weight; 11 lbs  4 oz          Label factor (answer) _____ kg
2. Determine the appropriate conversions.

Memorized conversions:

1 lb = 16 oz   or  $\dfrac{1 \text{ lb}}{16 \text{ oz}}$   or  $\dfrac{16 \text{ oz}}{1 \text{ lb}}$       1 kg = 2.2 lbs   or  $\dfrac{1 \text{ kg}}{2.2 \text{ lbs}}$   or  $\dfrac{2.2 \text{ lbs}}{1 \text{ kg}}$

3. Arrange the problem so that each label (unit of measurement) not wanted in the answer can be canceled by its placement as a numerator and a consecutive denominator.

4. Cancel unwanted labels (units of measurement) and circle all remaining label factors (answer).

| Step 1 | Step 2 | Step 3 |
|---|---|---|
| $\dfrac{4 \text{ oz}}{1} \text{ X } \dfrac{1 \text{ lb}}{16 \text{ oz}} = 0.25 \text{ lb}$ | Add<br>11.00 lbs<br>+ 0.25 lbs<br>11.25 lbs | $\dfrac{11.25 \text{ lbs}}{1} \text{ X } \dfrac{1 \text{ kg}}{2.2 \text{ lb}} = $ _____ kg |

5. Reduce numbers to lowest terms.

Not necessary

6. Multiply across the numerators. Multiply across the denominators. Divide the total numerator by the total denominator, creating a whole number or a number with a decimal point as the answer.

$$\frac{11.25}{1} \text{ X } \frac{1 \text{ kg}}{2.2} = \frac{11.25}{2.2} = 5.11 \text{ kg}$$

■ **In summary, 11 lbs. 4 oz equals 5.11 kg.**

**Note:** *Look at the answer, and ask is this answer reasonable? If it is not, check the numbers and recalculate.*

Once the infant's weight is converted from pounds to kilograms, it is usually written on the Kardex so that future drug calculations can be done using kilograms.

# Method: Dimensional Analysis
# Safe Dosage Calculation

Consult a reference for the safe dosage range. According to the Harriet Lane Handbook, the safe dosage range for erythromycin is 30 - 50 mg/kg/24 hours divided every 6 hours.

## B. What is the safe single dosage range for this infant?

*The physician's order is Ilosone (erythromycin) 62.5 mg po q6h. Is this dosage safe?*

The infant weighs 5.11 kg. Identify the label factor (units in the answer) and use as many conversions as you need to end up with that answer.

Conversion

Starting factor maximum dose: 50 mg/ kg/ day or $\dfrac{50 \text{ mg}}{1 \text{ kg x day}}$ or $\dfrac{1 \text{kg x day}}{50 \text{ mg}}$ $\quad \dfrac{1 \text{ dose}}{6 \text{ h}} \text{ X } \dfrac{24 \text{ h}}{1 \text{ day}} = 4 \dfrac{\text{doses}}{\text{day}}$

Label factor (answer) $\dfrac{\text{mg}}{\text{dose}}$

$$\dfrac{50 \text{ mg}}{\text{kg x day}} \text{ X } \dfrac{1 \text{ day}}{4 \text{ doses}} \text{ X } \dfrac{5.11 \text{ kg}}{1} = \underline{\qquad} \dfrac{\text{mg}}{\text{dose}}$$

$$\dfrac{50 \text{ x } 5.11}{4} \text{ X } \dfrac{255.5}{4} = 63.88 \dfrac{\text{mg}}{\text{dose}} \text{ (maximum dose)}$$

Starting factor minimum dose: 30 mg/ kg/ day

$$\dfrac{30 \text{ mg}}{\text{kg x day}} \text{ X } \dfrac{1 \text{ day}}{4 \text{ doses}} \text{ X } \dfrac{5.11 \text{ kg}}{1} = \underline{\qquad} \dfrac{\text{mg}}{\text{dose}}$$

$$\dfrac{30 \text{ x } 5.11}{4} = \dfrac{153.3}{4} = 38.33 \dfrac{\text{mg}}{\text{dose}} \text{ (minimum dose)}$$

Answer: Safe and therapeutic dosage range is 38.33 mg to 63.88 mg every 6 hours

## C. Is the ordered dosage within the safe range?

Answer:  Yes  62 .5 mg falls within the safe range.

## D. How many mg should be given per dosage?

Answer: 62.5 mg

## E. What route should the ordered medication be given?

Answer: po or by mouth

**F. The physician orders Ilosone (erythromycin) 62.5 mg, po q6h for a 11 lb 4 oz infant. How many mL of medication should be drawn into the syringe?**

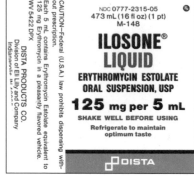

1. Identify starting factor and label factor.
Starting factor (order) 62.5 mg          Label factor (answer) mL

2. Identify the appropriate conversion.
Look at the medication label 125 mg = 5 mL or $\dfrac{125\ mg}{5\ mL}$ or $\dfrac{5\ mL}{125\ mg}$

No memorized conversion needed.

3. Arrange the problem so that each label (unit of measurement) not wanted in the answer can be canceled by its placement as a numerator and a consecutive denominator.

Starting factor (order) 62.5 mg          Label factor (answer) _____mL

$$\frac{62.5\ mg}{1} \times \frac{5\ mL}{125\ mg} = \text{_____ mL}$$

4. Cancel unwanted labels (units of measurement) and circle all remaining label factors (answer).

$$\frac{62.5\ \cancel{mg}}{1} \times \frac{5\ \boxed{mL}}{125\ \cancel{mg}} = \text{_____ mL}$$

5. Reduce numbers to lowest terms.

$$\frac{62.5}{1} \times \frac{\overset{1}{\cancel{5}}\ \boxed{mL}}{\underset{25}{\cancel{125}}} = \text{_____ mL}$$

6. Multiply across the numerators. Multiply across the denominators. Divide the total numerators by the total denominator, creating a whole number or a number with a decimal point as the answer.

$$\frac{62.5}{1} \times \frac{1\ \boxed{mL}}{25} = \frac{62.5}{25} = 2.5\ mL$$

■ In summary, Ilosone 62. 5 mg = 2.5 mL. Give 2.5 mL.

**Note:** *Look at the answer and ask is this answer reasonable. If it is not check the numbers and recalculate.*

**G. Calculate the answer in teaspoons instead of mL.**

■ Starting factor (order) 62.5 mg          Label factor (answer) _____tsp

Memorized conversion 1 tsp = 5 mL

conversion   drug label      order
$$\frac{1\ \boxed{tsp}}{\cancel{5}\ \cancel{mL}} \times \frac{\overset{1}{\cancel{5}}\ \cancel{mL}}{125\ \cancel{mg}} \times \frac{62.5\ \cancel{mg}}{1} = \frac{62.5}{125} = 0.5\ tsp$$

## H. Would the teaspoon measurement be practical?

Answer: Yes

Do practice problems 1-10 on rounding off on page 115 and then problems 11-20 starting on page 120 in chapter 7. Use the back cover to look up conversion factors if not memorized.

*Sample Problem*

# Method: Dimensional Analysis
# Pediatric Parenteral Administration

See chapter eight for more information about intravenous infusion rates.

*The physician orders Kefurox (cefuroxime) 350 mg IV q8h. The 10 month old infant weighs 16 lbs, 8 Oz. The nurse adds 3.6 mL of diluent to the vial.*

## A. Convert ounces to pounds
Step 1 convert ounces to pounds

Step 1

$$\frac{\overset{1}{\cancel{8\,oz}}}{1} \times \frac{1\,\cancel{lb}}{\underset{2}{\cancel{16\,oz}}} = 0.5\,lb$$

Step 2

Add
16.00
+ 0.5
16.5 lbs

## B. What is the safe single dosage range for this infant?

Consult a reference for the safe dosage range. The Harriet Lane Handbook states that the safe dosage for cefuroxime in infants and children is 75 - 150 mg/kg/24 hours divided every 8 hours.

**Note:** *This example uses the infant's weight in pounds.*

Identify starting factor and label factor.

Starting factor for maximum dose: 150 mg/kg/day

Label factor (answer) $\dfrac{mg}{dose}$

Identify the appropriate conversion.

Memorized conversion 1 kg = 2.2 lb

$$\frac{1\,\cancel{dose}}{\underset{1}{\cancel{8\,h}}} \times \frac{\overset{3}{\cancel{24\,h}}}{1\,\cancel{day}} = 3\,\frac{doses}{day}$$

Arrange the problem so that each label (unit of measurement) not wanted in the answer can be canceled by its placement as a numerator and a consecutive denominator.

$$\frac{150 \text{ mg}}{\text{kg} \times \text{day}} \times \frac{1 \text{ day}}{3 \text{ doses}} \times \frac{1 \text{ kg}}{2.2 \text{ lbs}} \times \frac{16.5 \text{ lbs}}{1} = \underline{\hspace{1cm}} \frac{\text{mg}}{\text{dose}}$$

Cancel unwanted labels (units of measurement) and circle all remaining label factors (answer).

$$\frac{150 \text{ⓜⓖ}}{\text{k̶g̶} \times \text{d̶a̶y̶}} \times \frac{1 \text{ d̶a̶y̶}}{3 \text{ ⓓⓞⓢⓔⓢ}} \times \frac{1 \text{ k̶g̶}}{2.2 \text{ l̶b̶s̶}} \times \frac{16.5 \text{ l̶b̶s̶}}{1} = \underline{\hspace{1cm}} \frac{\text{mg}}{\text{dose}}$$

Reduce to lowest terms. Multiply across the numerators. Multiply across the denominators. Divide the total numerators by the total denominators, creating a whole number or a number with a decimal point as the answer.

$$\frac{\overset{50}{\cancel{150}} \times 16.5}{\underset{1}{\cancel{3}} \times 2.2} = \frac{825}{2.2} = 375 \frac{\text{mg}}{\text{dose}} = \text{safe maximum dose}$$

▪ Starting factor for minimum dose: 75 mg /day

Label factor (answer) $\dfrac{\text{mg}}{\text{dose}}$

Arrange the problem so that each label (unit of measurement) not wanted in the answer can be canceled by its placement as a numerator and a consecutive denominator.

$$\frac{75 \text{ mg}}{\text{kg} \times \text{day}} \times \frac{1 \text{ day}}{3 \text{ doses}} \times \frac{1 \text{ kg}}{2.2 \text{ lbs}} \times \frac{16.5 \text{ lbs}}{1} = \underline{\hspace{1cm}} \frac{\text{mg}}{\text{dose}}$$

Cancel unwanted labels (units of measurement) and circle all remaining label factors (answer).

$$\frac{75 \text{ⓜⓖ}}{\text{k̶g̶} \times \text{d̶a̶y̶}} \times \frac{1 \text{ d̶a̶y̶}}{3 \text{ ⓓⓞⓢⓔⓢ}} \times \frac{1 \text{ k̶g̶}}{2.2 \text{ l̶b̶s̶}} \times \frac{16.5 \text{ l̶b̶s̶}}{1} = \underline{\hspace{1cm}} \frac{\text{mg}}{\text{dose}}$$

Reduce to lowest terms. Multiply across the numerators. Multiply across the denominators. Divide the total numerator by the total denominator, creating a whole number or a number with a decimal point as the answer.

$$\frac{\overset{25}{\cancel{75}} \times 16.5}{\underset{1}{\cancel{3}} \times 2.2} = \frac{412.5}{2.2} = 187.5 \text{ or } 188 \frac{\text{mg}}{\text{dose}} = \text{safe minimum dose}$$

Answer: Safe dosage range is 188 - 375 mg every 8 hours.

## C. Is the ordered dosage within the safe range?

Answer: Yes. The ordered dosage of 350 mg q8h falls between 188 - 375 mg and is within the safe dosage range.

## D. How many mg should you give per dosage?

>   Answer: 350 mg

**Note:** *Give what is ordered unless it is unsafe. You may not change the amount of medication ordered without a physician's order.*

## E. What route should the ordered medication be given?

>   Answer: IV

**Note:** *Administer medications by route ordered. If there is a concern, you must make the appropriate checks. You may not change the route without a physician's order.*

**Note:** *It is essential that you know by which route a medication may be safely given. Also, you need to assure that the form of the medication that is available may be given by the route ordered. Read the label or package insert for this information.*

## F. How many mL of medication should be drawn up for IV use?

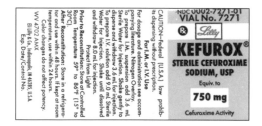

**Note:** *This label indicates that you can choose to dilute the medication in either 3.6 or 9 mL. Each amount will yield a different concentration. It is crucial that you know what the concentration is before determining how may mL would equal the ordered dosage. In this particular case, the nurse diluted the medication in 3.6 mL which yields 220 mg/mL. The strength of the medication then is 220 mg/mL as indicated in package insert.*

Starting factor 350 mg (order)          Label factor mL

$$\frac{350 \text{ mg}}{1} \times \frac{1 \text{ mL}}{220 \text{ mg}} = \underline{\hspace{1cm}} \text{mL} \quad \frac{35}{22} = 1.59 \text{ mL or } 1.6 \text{ mL rounding off}$$

>   Answer: 1.6 ml of Kefurox (cefuroxime) should be drawn into the syringe to have 350 mg.

**Note:** *If the medication is to be given IM, the nurse should give 1.6 mL. Since it is being given IV, the appropriate dilution and rate will need to be calculated.*

## G. What volume of fluid would be needed for maximum IV concentration?

(See Chapter 8 for more information on IV drug calculation.)

Determine the maximum concentration of cefuroxime to safely administer this medication IV.

**Note:** *There are established concentrations and rates for IV medication administration. The concentration and rate of administration must be followed to safely give an IV medication.*

Consult a reference or a pharmacist for recommended IV concentration and rate of administration. The Pediatric Dosage Handbook states cefuroxime intermittent infusion should be administered over 15-30 minutes at a concentration of 30 mg/mL.

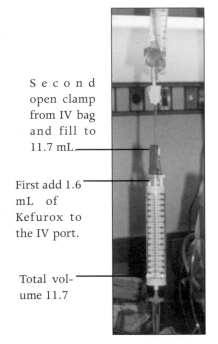

Second open clamp from IV bag and fill to 11.7 mL.

First add 1.6 mL of Kefurox to the IV port.

Total volume 11.7

Determine the maximum concentration to safely give cefuroxime 350 mg.

Starting factor 350 mg          Label factor mL

$$\frac{350 \overset{dose}{\cancel{mg}}}{1} X \frac{1 \overset{maximum\ conc.}{\cancel{mL}}}{30 \cancel{mg}} = \underline{\quad} mL \qquad \frac{\cancel{350}}{1} X \frac{1 \cancel{mL}}{\cancel{30}} = \frac{35}{3} = 11.7 \ mL$$

Answer: Dilute the 1.6 mL of cefuroxime to get a total volume of 11.7 mL

## H. What rate should the medication be delivered IV?

Determine the IV rate to safely give 350 mg of cefuroxime at 9 AM. Set up IV drip formula.

**Note:** *All children's IVs should be on a microdrip or a machine. The microdrip delivers 60 gtts per mL thus the drop factor would be 60.*

▪ Infusion rate at 15 minutes by microdrip tubing 60 gtt = 1 mL

Starting factor: $\dfrac{11.7 \ mL}{15 \ min}$          Label Factor: $\dfrac{gtt}{min}$

$$\frac{11.7 \ \cancel{mL}}{\underset{1}{\cancel{15}} \ \cancel{min}} X \frac{\overset{4}{\cancel{60}} \ \cancel{gtts}}{1 \ \cancel{mL}} = 46.8 \ \frac{gtt}{min} \quad \text{or} \ 47 \ gtt/min$$

▪ Infusion rate at 15 minutes by machine.

Starting factor: $\dfrac{11.7 \ mL}{15 \ min}$          Label Factor: $\dfrac{mL}{h}$

$$\frac{11.7 \ \cancel{mL}}{\underset{1}{\cancel{15}} \ \cancel{min}} X \frac{\overset{4}{\cancel{60}} \ \cancel{min}}{1 \ \cancel{h}} = 46.8 \ \frac{mL}{hr} \quad \text{or} \ 46.8 mL/h$$

**Problem H,** *cont.*

◼ Infusion rate at 30 minutes by microdrip tubing 60 gtt = 1 mL

$$\frac{11.7 \ \cancel{mL}}{\cancel{30} \ \cancel{\text{min}}} \ X \ \frac{\overset{2}{\cancel{60}} \ \cancel{\text{gtt}}}{1 \ \cancel{mL}} = 23.4 \ \frac{\text{gtt}}{\text{min}} \ \text{or} \ \ 23 \ \text{gtt/min}$$

◼ Infusion rate at 30 minutes by machine.

$$\frac{11.7 \ \cancel{mL}}{\cancel{30} \ \cancel{\text{min}}} \ X \ \frac{\overset{2}{\cancel{60}} \ \cancel{\text{min}}}{1 \ \cancel{h}} = 23.4 \ \frac{\text{mL}}{\text{h}} \ \text{or} \ \ 23.4 \ \text{mL/h}$$

   Answer: The 11.7 mL of diluted cefuroxime can be given at a rate of 23-47 gtts/min or mL/h.

**Note:** *The answer is the same for mL per hour and microdrops per minute (microdrip tubing 60 gtt = 1 mL). This is because 60 is placed in the same position for both problems. When using a microdrip tubing, drops are rounded to the nearest whole number. Whereas, pediatric pumps can measure to the nearest tenth.*

**Note:** *The stated volume may seem like a small amount to give IV. This is not unusual in the care of small infants and children. There is equipment which can deliver IV fluids in these volumes. The size of the child, physiological status, characteristics of the drug, and hospital policy will determine whether this amount will be given or if it will be further diluted. Unless indicated otherwise, this chapter will use the most concentrated of the usual concentration (most mg/mL) for calculating IV dilution. Usual dilution is frequently less concentrated than maximum concentration. IV medications should not be given in a volume less than maximum concentration indicates. Increasing the volume of diluent is acceptable practice.*

**Note:** *Pumps are set at mL per hour, which is the same rate as drops per minute. So, to give 23.4 gtt per minute, you set the pump at 23.4 mL/h. If you want to give 46.8 gtt per minute, you set the pump at 46.8 gtt per hour.*

Do practice problems 21-30 starting on page 131 in Chapter 7. Read pages 139-140 and do problems 31-35 found on page 141.

## Method: Dimensional Analysis
## Intravenous Infusion Rates Using a Pump, set at mL/h

*The physician orders 1 liter of D5W over 12 hours.*

Starting factor $\dfrac{1000 \text{ mL}}{12 \text{ h}}$        Label factor $\dfrac{\text{mL}}{\text{h}}$

$$\frac{1000 \text{ mL}}{12 \text{ h}} = 83 \frac{\text{mL}}{\text{h}}$$

Answer: Set the pump at 83 mL per hour to deliver 1000 mL over 12 hours.

## Method: Dimensional Analysis
## Calculation of IV Drip Rates Using Gravity Flow with Total Infusion Time Specified in the Order.

Drop factor 12 drops = 1 mL (found on the IV tubing package)
Memorized conversion 1 liter = 1000 mL

Starting factor $\dfrac{1000 \text{ mL}}{12 \text{ h}}$        Label factor $\underline{\hspace{1cm}} \dfrac{\text{gtts}}{\text{min}}$

$$\underset{\text{order}}{\frac{1000 \text{ m\!\!\!/L}}{12 \text{ \!\!/h}}} \quad \text{X} \quad \underset{\text{memorized conversion}}{\frac{1 \text{ \!\!/h}}{60 \text{ min}}} \quad \text{X} \quad \underset{\text{drop factor}}{\frac{12 \text{ gtts}}{1 \text{ m\!\!/L}}} = \underline{\hspace{1cm}} \frac{\text{gtts}}{\text{min}}$$

$$\frac{\overset{50}{\cancel{1000}}}{\cancel{12}} \text{ X } \frac{1}{\underset{3}{\cancel{60} \text{ min}}} \text{ X } \frac{\cancel{12} \text{ gtts}}{1} = \frac{50}{3} = \frac{16.6 \text{ gtts}}{\text{min}} = 17 \frac{\text{gtts}}{\text{min}}$$

Answer: Set the IV drop rate at 17 gtts/min to deliver 1 liter of D5W over 12 hours, using IV tubing that delivers 12 gtts/mL.

## Method: Dimensional Analysis
## Infusion Rate Specified in the Physician's Order

▮ *The physician orders Lactated Ringers 1000 mL at a rate of 75 mL per hour.*

The drop factor (from the IV package) is 15 gtts = 1mL.

Starting factor $\dfrac{75 \text{ mL}}{\text{h}}$      Label factor $\dfrac{\underline{\quad} \text{ gtts}}{\text{min}}$

$$\underset{\text{order}}{\dfrac{75 \text{ mL}}{1 \text{ h}}} \;\times\; \underset{\text{memorized conversion}}{\dfrac{1 \text{ h}}{60 \text{ min}}} \;\times\; \underset{\text{drop factor}}{\dfrac{15 \text{ gtts}}{1 \text{ mL}}} \;=\; \underline{\quad}\; \dfrac{\text{gtts}}{\text{min}}$$

$$\dfrac{75 \times \overset{1}{\cancel{15}}}{\underset{4}{\cancel{60}}} = 18.75 \,\dfrac{\text{gtts}}{\text{min}} = 19 \text{ gtts/min}$$

Answer: Set the IV drop rate at 19 drops per minute to deliver 75 mL per hour of Lactated Ringers, using IV tubing that delivers 15 gtts/mL.

## Method: Dimensional Analysis
## Intravenous Flow Rate for Piggyback Medication per Gravity.

The patient is to receive Zinacef 1 g in 50 mL D5W over 30 minutes.
Drop factor (from IV tubing package microdrip tubing) 60 gtts = 1 mL.

Starting factor $\dfrac{50 \text{ mL}}{30 \text{ min}}$      Label factor $\dfrac{\underline{\quad} \text{ gtts}}{\text{min}}$

$$\dfrac{50 \text{ mL}}{30 \text{ min}} \times \dfrac{60 \text{ gtts}}{1 \text{ mL}} = \underline{\quad}\; \dfrac{\text{gtts}}{\text{min}}$$

$$\dfrac{50 \times \overset{2}{\cancel{60}}}{\underset{1}{\cancel{30}}} = 100 \,\dfrac{\text{gtts}}{\text{min}}$$

Answer: Set the IV drop rate at 100 drops per minute to deliver 50 mL over 30 minutes, using microdrip tubing.

# Method: Dimensional Analysis
# Intravenous Flow Rate of a Piggyback Medication Using an Electronic Pump.

■ *The patient is to receive Zinacef 1 g in 50 mL D5W over 30 minutes.*

Starting factor $\dfrac{50\ \text{mL}}{30\ \text{min}}$ Label factor $\dfrac{_____\ \text{mL}}{\text{h}}$

$$\frac{50\ \cancel{\text{mL}}}{30\ \cancel{\text{min}}} \times \frac{60\ \cancel{\text{min}}}{1\ \cancel{\text{h}}} = \_\_\_\_\_\ \frac{\text{mL}}{\text{h}}$$

$$\frac{50 \times \overset{2}{\cancel{60}}}{\underset{1}{\cancel{30}}} = \frac{100\ \text{mL}}{\text{h}} = 100\ \frac{\text{mL}}{\text{h}}$$

Answer: Set the electronic pump at 100 mL per hour to deliver 50 mL over 30 minutes.

Note: *The answer is the same for mL/h as for gtts/min when using microdrop tubing (60 gtts = 1 mL). This is because 60 is placed in the same position in both problems.*

# Method: Dimensional Analysis
# Infusion Time

■ *1000 mL of D5W is to infuse at 125 mL/h. How many hours will it take for this liter of fluid to be completed?*

Starting factor 1000 mL   Label Factor _____h

$$\frac{1000\ \cancel{\text{mL}}}{1} \times \frac{1\ \cancel{\text{h}}}{125\ \cancel{\text{mL}}} = _____\text{h}$$

$$\frac{\overset{8}{\cancel{1000}}}{\underset{1}{\cancel{125}}} = 8\ \text{h}$$

Do practice problems 1-36 starting on page 159 in Chapter 8.

# Method: Dimensional Analysis
## Continuous Intravenous Infusion of a Drug Ordered Per Hour

■ *The physician orders heparin 800 units per hour. Read the label for the concentration of heparin.*

Heparin must always be given using an electronic pump. Calculate the flow rate in mL/h.

Starting factor $\dfrac{800\ u}{h}$  Label factor $\dfrac{mL}{h}$

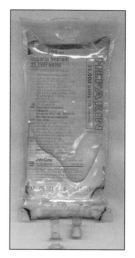

Dose on hand                Order
25,000 units of heparin in 250 mL    800 u = 1 hour

$$\frac{800\ \cancel{u}}{1\ \cancel{h}} \times \frac{250\ \cancel{mL}}{25,000\ \cancel{u}} = \underline{\qquad}\ \frac{mL}{h}$$

$$\frac{800}{1\ \cancel{h}} \times \frac{\overset{1}{\cancel{250}}\ \cancel{mL}}{\underset{100}{\cancel{25000}}} = \frac{800}{100} = 8\ \frac{mL}{h}$$

■ In summary, set the infusion pump at 8 mL/h which will deliver 800 units of heparin per hour.

# Method: Dimensional Analysis
## Determining the Units Per Hour With the Pump Set at a Given Rate Per Hour.

■ *The physician orders heparin 800 units per hour. The infusion pump is set at 8 mL/h. Is this the correct flow rate? Read the label from previous sample problem for the concentration of heparin.*

Starting factor $\dfrac{8\ mL}{h}$  Label factor $\dfrac{units}{h}$

$$\frac{8\ \cancel{mL}}{1\ \cancel{h}} \times \frac{\overset{100}{\cancel{25000}}\ \cancel{u}}{\underset{1}{\cancel{250}}\ \cancel{mL}} = \underline{\qquad}\ \frac{u}{h} \qquad\qquad \frac{8 \times 100}{1 \times 1} = 800\ \frac{units}{h}$$

■ In summary, an infusion rate of heparin at 8 mL/h is delivering heparin 800 units per hour. Yes, the flow rate is correct.

# Method: Dimensional Analysis
# Heparin Bolus

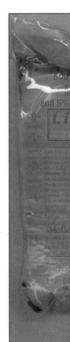

Give heparin 4000 u IV bolus now. Read the label.
Starting factor heparin   4000 u               Label factor mL

$$\overset{\text{order}}{\frac{4000 \,\cancel{u}}{1}} \times \overset{\text{dose on hand}}{\frac{1 \,\boxed{\text{mL}}}{5000 \,\cancel{u}}} = \underline{\hspace{1cm}} \text{mL} \qquad \frac{4}{5} = 0.8 \text{ mL}$$

**In summary, give 0.8 mL IV which equal 4000 units of heparin.**
Do problems 1-10 starting on page 176 in Chapter 9.

# Method: Dimensional Analysis
# Drugs Titrated Per Infusion Pump When Dosage Ordered mg
# Per Minute

*The physician orders Lidocaine 3 mg/min*

**Step I**
Determine the mg per mL of Lidocaine.
Starting factor $\dfrac{2\text{ g}}{500\text{ mL}}$          Label factor $\dfrac{\text{mg}}{\text{mL}}$

Conversions  1 g = 1000 mg    2 g = 500 mL
                  memorized              dose on hand

$$\frac{2\,\cancel{g}}{\underset{1}{\cancel{500}\,\boxed{\text{mL}}}} \times \frac{\overset{2}{\cancel{1000}\,\boxed{\text{mg}}}}{1\,\cancel{g}} = \frac{4 \text{ mg}}{\text{mL}}$$

*In summary, the concentration of Lidocaine is 4 mg/ mL.*

**Step II**
Determine the IV flow rate to deliver 3 mg/min

*The physician orders Lidocaine 3 mg/min*

Starting factor $\dfrac{3\text{ mg}}{\text{min}}$          Label factor $\dfrac{\text{mL}}{\text{h}}$

Conversions

| memorized conversion | order | dose on hand |
|---|---|---|
| 1 h = 60 mins | 1 min = 3 mg | 1 mL = 4 mg |

Sample Problem

**Lidocaine** *cont.*

$$\frac{\overset{15}{\cancel{60}\text{ min}}}{1\cancel{\text{h}}} \times \frac{3\cancel{\text{mg}}}{1\cancel{\text{min}}} \times \frac{1\cancel{\text{mL}}}{\cancel{4}\cancel{\text{mg}}} = \underline{\qquad}\frac{\text{mL}}{\text{h}} \quad \frac{15 \times 3}{1} = 45\,\frac{\text{mL}}{\text{h}}$$

With dimensional analysis, step 1 and step 2 can be combined as follows.

Identify the label factor (units in the answer) and then use as many conversions as you need to end up with that answer. Label factor $\frac{\text{mL}}{\text{h}}$

Combined problem with Lidocaine

$$\frac{500\,\cancel{\text{mL}}}{2\cancel{\text{g}}} \times \frac{1\cancel{\text{g}}}{1000\,\cancel{\text{mg}}} \times \frac{3\cancel{\text{mg}}}{1\cancel{\text{min}}} \times \frac{60\,\cancel{\text{min}}}{1\cancel{\text{h}}} = \underline{\qquad}\frac{\text{mL}}{\text{h}}$$

$$\frac{\overset{1}{\cancel{500}} \times 3 \times \overset{30}{\cancel{60}}}{2 \times \underset{\underset{1}{\cancel{2}}}{\cancel{1000}} \times 1} = \frac{90}{2} = 45\,\frac{\text{mL}}{\text{h}}$$

■ In summary, the pump set at 45 mL per hour will deliver Lidocaine 3 mg / min.

---

Sample Problem

# Method: Dimensional Analysis
# Checking Infusion Rate to Correlate with Correct Dosage.

■ *You find the infusion pump set at 45 mL/h. The patient is to receive lidocaine 3 mg per minute. Is this the correct flow rate? Read the label for the concentration of lidocaine.*

How many mg per minute is the patient receiving with an IV flow rate of 45 mL/h?

Starting factor $\frac{45\ \text{mL}}{\text{h}}$  Label factor $\frac{\text{mg}}{\text{min}}$

$$\frac{45\,\cancel{\text{mL}}}{1\cancel{\text{h}}} \times \frac{1\cancel{\text{h}}}{60\,\cancel{\text{min}}} \times \frac{2\cancel{\text{g}}}{500\,\cancel{\text{mL}}} \times \frac{1000\,\cancel{\text{mg}}}{1\cancel{\text{g}}} = \frac{45 \times 1 \times \overset{1}{\cancel{2}} \times \overset{2}{\cancel{1000}}}{1 \times \underset{30}{\cancel{60}} \times \underset{1}{\cancel{500}} \times 1} = \frac{90}{30} = 3\,\frac{\text{mg}}{\text{min}}$$

This problem could also be set up the following way.

**Note:** *With complex problems, it may be difficult to identify the starting factor. The sequence which you place the conversions is arbitrary, as long as the numerators and denominators are positioned correctly. Milligram is placed first as a numerator because that is the answer wanted. Other conversions are used to cancel units not wanted.*

$$\frac{1000\,\cancel{\text{mg}}}{1\cancel{\text{g}}} \times \frac{2\cancel{\text{g}}}{500\,\cancel{\text{mL}}} \times \frac{45\,\cancel{\text{mL}}}{1\cancel{\text{h}}} \times \frac{1\cancel{\text{h}}}{60\,\cancel{\text{min}}} = \frac{\overset{2}{\cancel{1000}} \times 2 \times \overset{3}{\cancel{45}} \times 1}{1 \times \underset{1}{\cancel{500}} \times 1 \times \underset{4}{\cancel{60}}} = \frac{2 \times 2 \times 3}{4} = \frac{12}{4} = 3\,\frac{\text{mg}}{\text{min}}$$

■ In summary, the pump set at 45 gtt per minute will deliver lidocaine 3 mg/min. Yes, this is the correct flow rate.

*Chapter Thirteen Dimensional Analysis* 247

# Method: Dimensional Analysis
# Drugs Titrated Per Infusion Pump When Dosage Ordered is Micrograms Per Minute.

*The physician orders nitroglycerin 5 mcg/min.*

Starting factor  $\dfrac{5 \text{ mcg}}{\text{min}}$     Label factor  $\dfrac{\text{mL}}{\text{h}}$

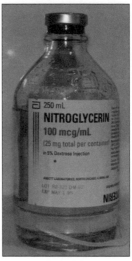

$$\frac{5 \text{ m\cancel{c}g}}{1 \text{ m\cancel{i}n}} \times \frac{\overset{3}{\cancel{60} \text{ m\cancel{i}n}}}{1 \text{ h}} \times \frac{1\,\cancel{\text{mL}}}{\underset{5}{\cancel{100} \text{ m\cancel{c}g}}} = \frac{15}{5} = 3 \frac{\text{mL}}{\text{h}}$$

order    conversion    dose on hand

**In summary, an IV infusion rate of 3 mL/h will deliver 5 mcg/min of nitro-glycerin with the concentration of 100 mcg/ml.**

**Note:** *Always check the bag for the concentration of the nitroglycerin per mL. Always double check the physician's order for the correct dosage. Always double check the calculations of the previous nurse. Although many medical centers use standard concentrations for ICU drugs, you can never assume that it is the standard concentration. Check the label.*

*The infusion pump is set at 3 mL/h. The physician order is nitroglycerin 5mcg/min. Is this the correct flow rate?*

Starting factor $\dfrac{3 \text{ mL}}{\text{h}}$     Label factor $\dfrac{\text{mcg}}{\text{min}}$

$$\frac{3 \text{ m\cancel{L}}}{1 \cancel{h}} \times \frac{1 \cancel{h}}{\cancel{60}\,\cancel{\text{min}}} \times \frac{\cancel{100}\,\cancel{\text{mcg}}}{1 \text{ m\cancel{L}}} = \frac{10 \times 3}{6} = 5 \frac{\text{mcg}}{\text{min}}$$

**In summary, Yes this is the correct flow rate. 3 mL/h is the correct IV infusion rate to deliver 5mcg/ min with the concentration of 100 mcg/mL of nitroglycerin.**

Do practice problems 1-5 on page 202 in Chapter 11.

# Method: Dimensional Analysis
# Drugs Titrated Per Infusion Pump at mL Per Hour Based Upon Micrograms Per Kilogram Per Minute

 *The physician orders: Titrate Nipride (nitroprusside) to keep the blood pressure less than 140 mm Hg systolic. Start the Nipride at 5 mcg/kg/min. The patient weighs 124 lbs.*

## Step I

Determine the concentration of the Nipride in $\dfrac{\text{mcg}}{\text{mL}}$

Starting factor $\dfrac{50 \text{ mg}}{250 \text{ mL}}$      Label factor $\dfrac{\text{mcg}}{\text{mL}}$

50 mg = 250 mL      1 mg = 1000 mcg
*dose on hand*      *memorized conversion*

$$\dfrac{50 \text{ m\!g}}{250 \text{ m\!L}} \times \dfrac{\overset{4}{1000} \text{ mcg}}{1 \text{ m\!g}} = 200 \dfrac{\text{mcg}}{\text{mL}}$$

## Step II

Determine the mcg/min that will deliver 5 mcg/kg/min.

Starting factor $\dfrac{5 \text{ mcg}}{\text{kg} \times \text{min}}$      Label factor $\dfrac{\text{mcg}}{\text{min}}$

$$\dfrac{5 \text{ mcg}}{1 \text{ k\!g} \times 1 \text{ min}} \times \dfrac{124 \text{ l\!b}}{1} \times \dfrac{1 \text{ k\!g}}{2.2 \text{ l\!b}} = \dfrac{124 \times 5}{2.2} = 282 \dfrac{\text{mcg}}{\text{min}}$$

## Step III

Determine the mL per hour that will deliver 5 mcg per kilogram per minute.

1 min = 282 mcg    200 mcg = 1 mL    60 min = 1 h
  *5 mcg/kg*        *dose on hand*    *memorized conversion*

Starting factor $\dfrac{282 \text{ mcg}}{1 \text{ min}}$      Label factor $\dfrac{\text{mL}}{\text{h}}$

$$\dfrac{282 \text{ m\!c\!g}}{1 \text{ m\!i\!n}} \times \dfrac{60 \text{ m\!i\!n}}{1 \text{ h}} \times \dfrac{1 \text{ mL}}{200 \text{ m\!c\!g}} = \dfrac{282 \times 6}{20} = 85 \dfrac{\text{mL}}{\text{h}}$$

**Note:** *This problem may be done as a combined problem. Identify the label factor (units in the answer) and then use as many conversions as needed to end up with that answer.*

## Combined Problem

Starting factor $\dfrac{5 \text{ mcg}}{\text{kg} \times 1 \text{ min}}$      Label factor $\dfrac{\text{mL}}{\text{h}}$

**Combined Problem,** *cont.*

order         weight    concentration

$$\frac{5 \text{ mcg}}{\text{kg} \times \text{min}} \times \frac{1 \text{ kg}}{2.2 \text{ lb}} \times \frac{124 \text{ lb}}{1} \times \frac{250 \text{ mL}}{50 \text{ mg}} \times \frac{1 \text{ mg}}{1000 \text{ mcg}} \times \frac{60 \text{ min}}{1 \text{ h}} = \frac{5 \times 124 \times 250 \times 60}{2.2 \times 50 \times 1000} = \frac{124 \times 6}{4 \times 2.2} = \frac{744}{8.8} = 84.6 \text{ or } 85 \frac{\text{mL}}{\text{h}}$$

*Sample Problem*

---

# Method: Dimensional Analysis
# Calculation of a constant for this patient for mcg/kg/min which is based on mL/h and mg/min.

Nipride 50 mg/ 250 mL     1 hour = 60 min    1 kg = 2.2 lbs    1000 mcg = 1 mg

CONSTANT                                              CONSTANT

$$\frac{? \text{ mL}}{1 \text{ h}} \times \left( \frac{1 \text{ h}}{60 \text{ min}} \times \frac{50 \text{ mg}}{250 \text{ mL}} \times \frac{1000 \text{ mcg}}{1 \text{ mg}} \times \frac{1}{124 \text{ lb}} \times \frac{2.2 \text{ lbs}}{1 \text{ kg}} \right) = \frac{50 \times 1000 \times 2.2}{60 \times 250 \quad 124} = \frac{5 \times 4 \times 2.2}{6 \times 124} = \frac{44}{744} = 0.059$$

$$0.059 \times \frac{\text{mL}}{\text{h}} = \underline{\phantom{xxxxx}} \frac{\text{mcg}}{\text{kg/min}}$$

*Sample Problem*

---

# Method: Dimensional Analysis
# Using the Constant to Determine $\dfrac{\text{mcg}}{\text{kg} \times \text{min}}$

As a shortcut, once the constant has been calculated for this patient, you can directly multiply it by each changing flow rate (mL/h) to obtain the answer.

**A. The patient's BP is 138 systolic and the Nipride has been decreased to 20 mL/h. How many mcg/kg/min is the patient receiving?**

$$0.059 \times 20 = 1.2 \quad \frac{\text{mcg}}{\text{kg} \times \text{min}}$$

**B. The patient's BP is 130 systolic and the Nipride has been decreased to 15 mL/h. How many mcg/kg/min is the patient receiving?**

$$0.059 \times 15 = 0.9 \quad \frac{\text{mcg}}{\text{kg} \times \text{min}}$$

Do practice problems 6-23, starting on page 205 in Chapter 11. Complete the Post Test starting on page 251.

# Post Test

## Chapter Two: Ratio Proportion

Include the units such as mL, capsule, table drop/min, and mL/h with your answer.

1. Mrs. Jones has been on Prozac (fluoxetine HCl) 20 mg PO qd in the morning for 4 weeks and has shown no sign of clinical improvement with the symptoms of depression. The doctor increases the Prozac to 30 mg po q AM.
   How supplied: Prozac 10 mg per capsule.

   Give? _____

2. Mr. Brown's blood sugar has been slightly elevated. The doctor orders Diabeta (glyburide) 5 mg po qd with breakfast.
   How supplied: Diabeta 2.5 mg per tablet.

   Give? _____

3. The doctor ordered Feldene (piroxicam) 20 mg po qd for Mrs. Nowakowski's osteoarthritis.
   How supplied: Feldene 10 mg per capsule.

   Give? _____

4. Mr. Burnam has asthma. The doctor ordered Proventil syrup (albuterol sulfate) 1.5 mg po q6h.
   How supplied: Proventil 2 mg per 5 mL.

   Give? _____

5. The doctor orders Procardia (nifedipine) XL 30 mg po qd.
   How supplied: a. Procardia 10 mg per capsule or b. Procardia 30 mg XL per capsule.

   Give?a. _____ or b. _____

6. Mrs. Jones is very restless. The physician orders Valium (diazepam) 2 mg IV push now.
   How supplied: diazepam 5 mg/mL for intramuscular or intravenous use.

   Give? _____

7. The doctor orders Demerol (meperidine) 75 mg IM q3h prn pain postoperatively for Mrs. Howland.
   How supplied: Demerol 100 mg/mL for intramuscular, subcutaneous, and intravenous use.

   Give? _____

8. The doctor orders Lanoxin (digoxin) 0.125 mg IV qd.
   How supplied: Lanoxin 0.5 mg per 2 mL.


   Give? _____

9. The doctor orders Dilaudid (hydromorphone) 0.25 mg IV now for a patient in the cath lab.
   How supplied: Dilaudid 2 mg/mL.


   Give? _____

10. The physician orders Torecan (thiethylperazine) 7.5 mg IM q8h prn for Sister Margaret's nausea.
    How supplied: Torecan 10 mg/2mL.


    Give? _____

## Chapter Four: Conversion From One System to Another

11. gr iii = _____ mg

12. 0.5 g = _____ mg

13. 78 kg = _____ lb

14. 300 mg = _____ mcg

15. 2 oz = _____ mL

## Chapter Five: Drug Calculations Requiring Conversions

16. The physician orders Dilaudid (hydromorphone) 4 mg po q4h prn pain.
    How supplied: Dilaudid 5 mg/tsp.


    Give? _____

17. The doctor orders atropine gr 1/150 IM preoperatively.
    How supplied: Atropine 0.4 mg/mL.


    Give? _____

18. Nipride (nitroprusside) 50 mg has been added to 250 mL of D5W.

    How many mcg have been added to 250 mL? _____

**Chapter Five** *cont.*

19. The doctor orders Aspirin gr XV suppository per rectum stat for a fever of 104.
    How supplied: Aspirin 625 mg/suppository.

    Give? _____

20. The physician orders morphine sulfate gr 1/6 SQ q4h prn pain.
    How supplied: morphine sulfate 10 mg/mL.

    Give? _____

## Chapter Six: Reconstitution of Powdered Drugs

21. The vial contains 5,000,000 units of penicillin G for injection. The vial label reads for preparation of solution: add 23 mL, 18 mL, 8 mL, or 3 mL diluent to provide 200,000 units, 250,000 units, 500,000 units, 1,000,000 units per mL respectively.

    To get 250,000 units per mL you would add _____ mL of normal saline.

22. The vial contains Vancocin 500 mg for intravenous use. The vial has been diluted with 10 mL of sterile water for injection. Vial reconstituted in this manner will contain 50 mg/mL.
    The doctor orders Vancocin 250 mg IV PB in 100 mL D5W.

    How many mL is necessary to give 250 mg of Vancocin? _____

23. The vial contains Kefzol 1 g.
    The package insert states:
    > 250 mg vial add 2 mL to get 125 mg/mL
    > 500 mg vial add 2 mL to get 225 mg/mL
    > 1 g vial add 2.5 mL to get 330 mg/mL

    How much diluent should be added to a 1 g vial? _____ to get 330 mg/mL

24. The vial contains ampicillin 1 g. The physician orders ampicillin 300 mg IM now. The vial is labeled that it was diluted for IM use with 3.5 mL of diluent resulting in 250 mg of ampicillin per mL.

    Give? _____

25. The vial contains penicillin G The label reads:
    potassium penicillin 1,000,000 units.

    |  | Add diluent | Conc. of Solution |
    |---|---|---|
    | 3/15 | 9.6 mL | 100,000 units/mL |
    |  | 4.4 mL | 300,000 units/mL |
    |  | 1.6 mL | 500,000 units/mL |

    It is 6 PM March 15 and the doctor has ordered penicillin G 200,000 units IM now.

    Give? _____

## Chapter Seven: Pediatric Drug Calculation

26. The physician orders Valium (diazepam) 6 mg, po, q6h PRN for restlessness. The child weighs 66 lbs. *The Harriet Lane Handbook* states that the safe dose for diazepam when given for sedation is 0.12 - 0.8 mg/kg 24 hours divided every 6-8 hours.

    Label reads: Diazepam 5 mg/5 mL
    a.   What is the child's weight in kg?                                                  _____
    b.   What is the safe 24 hour dosage range for this child?                  _____
    c.   What is the safe single dosage range?                                        _____
    d.   Is the dosage ordered within a safe range?                                 _____
    e.   How many mg should the nurse give per dose?                          _____
    f.   What route should the medication be given?                              _____
    g.   How many mL of medication should be drawn up?                    _____
    h.   How many teaspoons would equal the ordered amount?             _____
    i.   Would the teaspoon measurement be practical?                         _____

27. The physician orders Rocephin (ceftriaxone), 590 mg, IV, q12h. The child weighs 25 lbs 15 oz. *The Harriet Lane Handbook* states that the safe dose for infants and children with meningitis is 100 mg/kg/24 hours divided every 12 hours. The *Pediatric Dosage Handbook* states that the safe intermittent IV concentration for ceftriaxone is 40 mg/mL and it would be given over 10-30 minutes. The nurse adds 3.6 mL of diluent to the vial.

    Label reads: Ceftriaxone 1 g/vial. Add 3.6 mL diluent to yield 250 mg/mL
    a.   What is the child's weight in kg?                                                  _____
    b.   What is the safe 24 hour dosage range for this child?                  _____
    c.   What is the safe single dosage range?                                        _____
    d.   Is the dosage ordered within a safe range?                                 _____
    e.   How many mg should the nurse give per dose?                          _____
    f.   What route should the medication be given?                              _____
    g.   How many mL of medication should be drawn up for IM use?    _____
    h.   What volume of fluid would be needed for maximum IV
         concentration?                                                                            _____
    i.   What rate should the medication be delivered IV?                      _____

28. The physician orders Tylenol (acetaminophen), 90 mg, po, q4h PRN for temp above 101. The child weighs 16 lbs. The *Harriet Lane Handbook* states that the safe dose for acetaminophen is 10-15 mg/kg/ dose given every 4 hours.

    Label reads: Acetaminophen 160 mg/5 cc
    a.   What is the child's weight in kg?                                                  _____
    b.   What is the safe 24 hour dosage range for this child?                  _____
    c.   What is the safe single dosage range?                                        _____
    d.   Is the dosage ordered within a safe range?                                 _____
    e.   How many mg should the nurse give per dose?                          _____
    f.   What route should the medication be given?                              _____
    g.   How many mL of medication should be drawn up?                    _____
    h.   How many teaspoons would equal the ordered amount?             _____
    i.   Would the teaspoon measurement be practicial?                        _____

**Chapter Seven** *cont.*

29. The physician orders Claforan (cefotaxime) 480 mg, IV, q8h. The child weighs 15 lbs 14 oz. *The Harriet Lane Handbook* states that the safe dosage for cefotaxime is 100-200 mg/kg/24 hours divided every 6-8 hours. The *Pediatric Dosage Handbook* states that the safe intermittent IV concentration fo cefotaxime is 20-60 mg/mL and it would be given over 15-30 minutes. The nurse adds 2 mL of diluent to the vial.

    Label reads: Cefotaxime 500 mg/vial. Add 2 mL of diluent to yield 230 mg/mL
    a. What is the child's weight in kg? _____
    b. What is the safe 24 hour dosage range for this child? _____
    c. What is the safe single dosage range? _____
    d. Is the dosage ordered within a safe range? _____
    e. How many mg should the nurse give per dose? _____
    f. What route should the medication be given? _____
    g. How many mL of medication should be drawn up for IM use? _____
    h. What volume of fluid would be needed for maximum IV concentration? _____
    i. What rate should the medication be delivered IV? _____

30. The physician orders Lanoxin (digoxin) 75 mcg, po, bid. The child is 9 years old and weighs 33 lbs 8 oz. *The Harriet Lane Handbook* states that the safe dose for digoxin in a child 2-10 years of age is 8-10 mcg/kg/24 hours given bid.

    Label reads: Digoxin 50 mcg/mL
    a. What is the child's weight in kg? _____
    b. What is the safe 24 hour dosage range for this child? _____
    c. What is the safe single dosage range? _____
    d. Is the dosage ordered within a safe range? _____
    e. How many mcg should the nurse give per dose? _____
    f. What route should the medication be given? _____
    g. How many mL of medication should be drawn up? _____

## Chapter Eight: Intravenous Infusion Rates

31. The physician orders 1 unit of packed cells over three hours. The unit contain 220 mL. The drop factor is 10 drops = 1 mL.

    Calculate the flow rate in drops per minute. _____

32. The physician orders 500 mL of lipids over 10 hours. An electronic infusion pump is used.

    Calculate the flow rate in mL per hour. _____

33. The physician orders 2000 mL over D5LR over 16 hours. Gravity flow is used for this day surgery patient. Drop factor: 20 drops = 1 mL.

    Calculate the flow rate in drops per minute. _____

34. The physician orders a TKO IV at 10 mL per hour.
    Drop factor: 60 drops = 1 mL.


    Calculate the flow rate in drops per minute. _____

35. The physician orders 1,000 mL D5 0.45 over 12 hours.
    Drop factor: 15 drops = 1 mL.

    a.   Calculate the flow rate in drops per min. _____

    b.   Calculate the electric flow rate in mL per hour. _____

## Chapter Nine: Heparin

36. The physician orders heparin 3,000 units SQ q8h.
    How supplied: Heparin 10,000 units/ mL.



    Give? _____

37. The physician orders heparin 8,000 units IV now.
    How supplied: Heparin 20,000 units/mL



    Give? _____

38. The physician orders a heparin drip at 900 units per hour.
    Concentration of heparin is: 25,000 units in 250 mL.



    Calculate the electronic pump flow rate in mL/h. _____

39. The physician orders a heparin drip at 600 units per hour.
    Concentration of heparin is 25,000 units in 250 mL.



    Calculate the electronic pump flow rate in mL/h. _____

40. The physician orders a heparin drip at 700 units per hour.
    Concentration of heparin is: 25,000 units in 500 mL.



    Calculate the electronic pump flow rate in mL/h. _____

**Post Test**

**Chapter Ten: Insulin**

41. The physician orders NPH 6 units of insulin SQ q AM.
    How supplied: NPH 100 units/mL

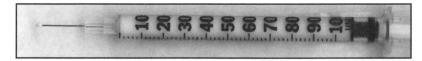

    Draw an arrow to the corrrect number of units.

42. The physician orders NPH 28 units of insulin SQ q AM.
    How supplied: NPH 100 units/mL

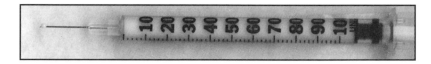

    Draw an arrow to the corrrect number of units.

43. The physician orders 15 units of Regular insulin now.
    How supplied: 100 units/mL

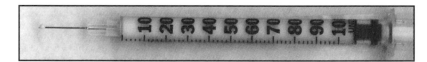

    Draw an arrow to the correct number of units.

44. The physician orders NPH insulin 16 units and regular insulin 5 units q AM before breakfast.
    How supplied: NPH 100 units/mL. Regular 100 units/mL
    a. Which insulin is drawn first? _____

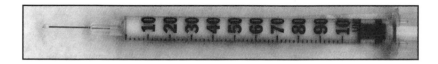

    b. Draw an arrow to the corrrect measurement for each insulin.

45. The physician orders an insulin drip at 9 units per hour. The concentration of insulin is: 50 units regular insulin in 100 mL of NS.

    Calculate the electronic infusion pump in mL per hour. _____

## Chapter Eleven: Titrated Drugs Used in Critical Care

46. The physician orders a Dobutrex (dobutamine) drip at 5 mcg/kg/min. The patient weighs 202 pounds. The concentration of dobutamine is 500 mg in 250 mL of D5W.

    Calculate the electronic pump infusion rate in mL/h. _____

47. The physician orders a lidocaine drip at 3 mg per minute. The concentration of lidocaine is: 2 g in 500 mL of D5W.

    Calculate the electronic pump infusion rate in mL/h. _____

48. You check the dopamine drip and it is infusing at 15 mL/h. The patient weighs 58 kg. The concentration of dopamine is 800 mg/500 mL D5W.

    How many mcg/kg/min of dopamine is the patient receiving? _____

49. The patient is on a nitroglycerin drip for chest pain. You check the drip and it is infusing at 10 mL/h. The concentration of nitroglycerin is 50 mg/250 mL of D5W.

    How many mcg per minute is the patient receiving? _____

50. The physician orders an Inocor (amrinone) drip at 5 mcg/kg/min. The patient weighs 120 pounds. The concentration of Inocor is 100 mg/100 mL of NS.

    Calculate the electronic pump infusion rate in mL/h. _____

## Post Test

## Chapter Twelve: Community Nursing and the Elderly

51. The physician orders (5%) solution of betadine for a foot soak for your home care patient. Prepare 500 mL of a 5% Betadine solution. The stock solution is Betadine 10%. The diluent is normal saline. How much betadine do you need and how much normal saline do you need?

    a. V1—Final volume you want to prepare?                                    _____
    b. C1—Concentration of the solution you wish to prepare?                   _____
    c. V2—Volume of stock solution you will need for dilution?                 _____
    d. C2—Concentration of the stock solution you will use?                    _____
    e. What is the unknown and what is the formula?                            _____
    f. How much stock solution is needed?                                      _____
    g. How much diluent is needed? (V1-V2)                                     _____

52. You have only 50 mL of betadine 10% stock solution left in the bottle. You wish to prepare a ¼ strength or 2.5% strength solution from the 50 mL of betadine using normal saline as the diluent.

    a. V1—Final volume you want to prepare?                                    _____
    b. C1—Concentration of the solution you wish to prepare?                   _____
    c. V2—Volume of stock solution you will need for dilution?                 _____
    d. C2—Concentration of the stock solution you will use?                    _____
    e. What is the unknown and what is the formula?                            _____
    f. What is the final volume (V1) needed to make a 2.5% solution from 50 mL of betadine?   _____
    g. How much diluent is needed? (V1-V2)                                     _____

53. You wish to prepare 800 mL of a 0.1% solution for a vinegar douche. Stock solution of vinegar is 5% acidity. Diluent is tap water.

    a. V1—Final volume you want to prepare?                                    _____
    b. C1—Concentration of the solution you wish to prepare?                   _____
    c. V2—Volume of stock solution you will need for dilution?                 _____
    d. C2—Concentration of the stock solution you will use?                    _____
    e. What is the unknown and what is the formula?                            _____
    f. How much stock solution (V2) is needed?                                 _____
    g. How much diluent is needed? (V1-V2)                                     _____

54. Mr. Wray is a 55 year old male who weighs 82 kg. This is close to his ideal body weight. His serum creatinine is 1 mg/dl. Using the Cockroft-Gault formula calculate the estimated creatinine clearance. _____

55. Mr. Peterschmidt is a 70 year old male patient who weight 71 kg. This is his ideal body weight. His serum creatinine is 1.7 mg/dl. Using the Cockroft-Gault formula calculate the estimated creatinine clearance. _____

56. Ms. Davis is a 40 year old female who weighs 55 kg. This is her ideal body weight. Her serum creatinine is 0.7 mg/dl. Using the Cockroft-Gault formula calculate the estimated creatinine clearance. _____

57. Ms. Bado is a 89 year old female and weighs 60 kg. This is her ideal body weight. Her serum creatinine is 1.2 mg/dl. Using the Cockroft-Gault formula calculate the estimated creatinine clearance. _____

58. Mr. Jones is 65 years old and weighs 100 kg. However his ideal body weight is 70 kg. Calculate the dose adjusted weight. _____

59. Mr. Blake has a post operative would infection. He weighs 150 lbs or 68.2 kg. The physician orders gentamicin 50 mg IV PB q 8 h. Mr. Blake is started on the gentamicin in the hospital and was then discharged home to continue IV therapy with home health care nursing. The drug handbook states that the IV dose of gentamicin is 1.5-2 mg per kg divided in three doses.
Is gentamicin 40 mg IV PB q 8 h safe? _____

60. The pharmacy has delivered a 24 hour supply of gentamicin 40 mg in 100 mL of D5W to Mr. Blake's home. The home heath nurse draws the trough level of gentamicin at 1330 which is 30 minutes before the 1400 gentamicin is due. A peak level of gentamicin (serum specimen) is ordered following the 2 P.M. (1400) dose of gentamicin. There is a IV pump to deliver the gentamicin. To get an accurate peak level the gentamicin must be given over exactly 30 minutes and a peak level drawn 30 minutes following the infusion. What is the correct IV infusion rate? _____

61. Mr. Blake's peak gentamicin level is **7 mcg/mL** and his trough level is **1 mcg/mL**.

**Note:** The Geriatric Dosage Handbook *states the therapeutic peak level is 4-8 mcg/mL and the therapeutic trough level is <2mch/mL. The MIC (minimum inhibitory concentration) reported from the lab indicates 0.5 mcg/mL is sufficient to inhibit bacterial growth.*

a. Does Mr. Blake's peak level fall within the therapeutic range?      _____
b. Does the trough level fall within the therapeutic range?      _____
c. Does the trough level fall above the MIC?      _____

62. Ms. Beach, a 68 year old patient, is on a maintenance dose of digoxin 0.25 mg qd. A digoxin blood level was obtained 8 hours after she last took her morning digoxin.

**Note:** *The normal therapeutic range for digoxin is 0.5-2 ng/mL.*

The home health nurse reviews the lab report for the digoxin level and finds Ms. Beach's level to be 0.6 ng/mL.

Is the maintenance dose of digoxin 0.25 mg qd maintaining
the digoxin level within the therapeutic range?      _____

## Post Test Answers: 1-62

Chapter Two
1.  3 capsules
2.  2 tablets
3.  2 tablets
4.  3.75 mL
5.  b
6.  0.4 mL
7.  0.75 mL
8.  0.5 mL
9.  0.125 mL
10. 1.5 mL

Chapter Four
ll. 180 mg
12. 500 mg
13. 171.6 lbs
14. 300,000 mcg
15. 60 mL

Chapter Five
16. 4 mL
17. 1 mL
18. 50,000 mcg
19. 1.5 suppository
20. 1 mL

Chapter Six
21. 18 mL
22. 5 mL
23. 2.5 mL
24. 1.2 mL
25. 2 mL

Chapter Seven
26.
a.  30 kg
b.  3.6-24 mg/24 hrs
c.  0.9-6 mg per dose
d.  Yes
e.  6 mg
f.  Oral
g.  6 mL
h.  1.2 tsp. or 1 1/5 tsp.
i.  No, measurement in a syringe would be more appropriate

Chapter Seven, *cont.*
27.
a.  11.79 kg
b.  1179 mg/24 hrs
c.  589.5 mg/dose

d.  Yes
e.  590 mg
f.  IV
g.  2.4 mL
h.  14.8 mL
i.  29.6 - 88.8 mL/h or gtts/min

28.
a.  7.27 kg
b.  Not appropriate since recommendation is per dose
c.  72.7 - 109.05 mg/dose
d.  Yes
e.  90 mg
f.  Oral
g.  2.8 mL
h.  0.56
i.  No, measurement in a syringe would be more appropriate.

29.
a.  7.22 kg
b.  722 - 1444 mg/24 hrs
c.  240.67 - 481.33 mg/dose
d.  Yes
e.  480 mg
f.  IV
g.  2.1 mL
h.  8 mL
i.  16 - 32 mL

30.
a.  15.23 kg
b.  121.84 - 152.3 mg/24 hrs
c.  60.92 - 76.15 mg/dose
d.  Yes
e.  75 mcg
f.  Oral
g.  1.5 mL

Chapter Eight
31. 12 drops/min
32. 50 mL/h
33. 42 drops/min
34. 10 drops/min
35. a.  21 drops/min
    b.  83 mL/h

Chapter Nine
36. 0.3 mL
37. 0.4 mL

38. 9 mL/h
39. 6 mL/h
40. 14 mL/h

Chapter Ten
41. 6 unit marker
42. 28 units marker
43. 15 unit marker
44. a.  Regular insulin
    b.  5 unit marker for Regular and 16 unit marker for NPH. Total = 21.
45. 18 mL/h

Chapter Eleven
46. 14 mL/h
47. 45 mL/h
48. 6.9 mcg/kg/min
49. 33 mcg/min
50. 17 mL/h

Chapter Twelve
51. a.  500 mL
    b.  5%
    c.  unknown
    d.  10%
    e.  $V_2 = \dfrac{V_1 \times C_1}{C_2}$
    f.  250 mL betadine
    g.  250 mL normal saline

52. a.  unknown
    b.  2.5%
    c.  50 mL
    d.  10%
    e.  $V_1 = \dfrac{V_2 \times C_2}{C_1}$
    f.  200 mL
    g.  150 mL normal saline

53. a.  800 mL
    b.  0.1%
    c.  unknown
    d.  5%
    e.  $V_2 = \dfrac{V_1 \times C_1}{C_2}$
    f.  16 mL vinegar
    g.  784 mL tap water

54. The estimated creatinine clearance is 97 mL/minute.

**Answers,** *cont.*

55. The estimated creatinine clearance is 41 mL/minute.

56. The estimated creatinine clearance is 93 mL/minute.

57. The estimated creatinine clearance is 30 mL/minute.

58. The adjusted weight is 82 kg.

59. Yes, the safe range for a patient weighing 68.2 kg is 34.1-45.5 mg.

60. 200 mL/h

61. a.  Yes
    b.  Yes
    c.  Yes

62. Yes

**14**

Chapter Fourteen

# Basic Math Review

# Introduction

This chapter presents a basic review of Roman numerals, addition, subtraction, multiplication and division of decimals and fractions. It also discusses ratios, percents, and equivalents for decimals, fractions, ratios and percents.

After completing this chapter you will be able to:

1. Recognize the Arabic values of Roman Numerals
2. Add, subtract, multiply and divide decimals
3. Add, subtract, multiply and divide fractions
4. Find equivalents of decimals, fractions, ratios and percents.

## Take the pretest before doing the chapter.

The pretest will determine if you need to review this chapter. If you miss more than one in each section, of the pretest, you need to review the entire chapter.

# Pretest

## Add the decimals

1. $2.40 + 0.4 + 1.03 =$

2. $0.5 + 0.5 + 0.5 =$

3. $5.3 + 2.6 + 0.09 =$

## Subtract the decimals

4. $1.9 - 0.08 =$

5. $3.95 - 0.45 =$

6. $48.638 - 37.796 =$

## Multiply the decimals

7. $2.14 \times 0.9 =$

8. $3.5 \times 1.2 =$

9. $8.5 \times 0.96 =$

## Divide the decimals

10. $0.30 \div 25 =$

11. $8.4 \div 0.7 =$

12. $3.0 \div 25 =$

## Which of the decimals has the highest value?

13. *a.* 3.55    *b.* 2.95    *c.* 3.9

14. *a.* 4.75    *b.* 7.6    *c.* 6.2

15. *a.* 0.22    *b.* 0.23    *c.* 0.24

# Pretest

**Add the fractions**

16. $\dfrac{3}{4} + \dfrac{4}{5} =$

17. $\dfrac{1}{4} + 2\dfrac{5}{8} =$

18. $\dfrac{1}{3} + 2\dfrac{3}{8} + \dfrac{2}{3} =$

**Subtract the fractions**

19. $\dfrac{3}{4} - \dfrac{2}{9} =$

20. $\dfrac{2}{3} - \dfrac{1}{2} =$

21. $2\dfrac{1}{4} - \dfrac{1}{3} =$

**Multiply the fractions**

22. $\dfrac{7}{8} \times \dfrac{2}{3} =$

23. $\dfrac{23}{4} \times \dfrac{1}{3} =$

24. $\dfrac{1}{6} \times \dfrac{2}{3} =$

# Pretest

**Divide the fractions**

25. $\dfrac{1}{10} \div \dfrac{1}{6} =$

26. $\dfrac{3}{4} \div \dfrac{2}{3} =$

27. $\dfrac{4}{5} \div \dfrac{5}{9} =$

**Find the equivalents of the following percents.**

| | percent | decimal | ratio | fraction |
|---|---|---|---|---|
| 28. | 20% | _____ | _____ | _____ |
| 29. | 2.5% | _____ | _____ | _____ |
| 30. | 40% | _____ | _____ | _____ |

**Solve for X**

31. $\dfrac{30}{60} = \dfrac{10}{X}$     X = _____

32. $\dfrac{1}{8} = \dfrac{12}{X}$     X = _____

33. $\dfrac{50}{2} = \dfrac{25}{X}$     X = _____

# Pretest Answers

1. 3.83    2. 1.5    3. 7.99    4. 1.82    5. 3.5

6. 10.842    7. 1.926    8. 4.2    9. 8.16    10. 0.012

11. 12    12. 0.12    13. *c* 3.9    14. *b* 7.6    15. 0.24

16. $1\frac{11}{20}$    17. $2\frac{7}{8}$    18. $3\frac{3}{8}$    19. $\frac{19}{36}$    20. $\frac{1}{6}$

21. $1\frac{11}{12}$    22. $\frac{7}{12}$    23. $1\frac{11}{12}$    24. $\frac{1}{9}$    25. $\frac{3}{5}$

26. 1.125 or $1\frac{1}{8}$    27. $1\frac{11}{25}$

| | percent | decimal | ratio | fraction |
|---|---|---|---|---|
| 28. | 20% | 0.2 | 1:5 | $\frac{1}{5}$ |
| 29. | 2.5% | 0.025 | 1:40 | $\frac{1}{40}$ |
| 30. | 40% | 0.4 | 2:5 | $\frac{2}{5}$ |

31. 20

32. 96

33. 1

The following is a list of the question numbers in the pretest and the page numbers in Chapter 12 that explain the concepts.

Pretest questions 1-15 on Decimals. Refer to Chapter 12, pages 229-234.
Pretest questions 16-27 on Fractions. Refer to Chapter 12, pages 235-242.
Pretest questions 28-33 on Ratios. Refer to Chapter 12, pages 243-246.

# Roman Numerals

The use of Roman numerals dates back to ancient times when those in the medical profession used its symbols for record keeping. Modern medicine has retained some of that tradition by using Roman numerals in prescribing medications. The Roman system uses letters to designate numbers.

## Roman Numerals and Equivalents

| Roman Numeral | Arabic Equivalent | Roman Numeral | Arabic Equivalent |
|---|---|---|---|
| ss | 1/2 | ix | 9 |
| i | 1 | x | 10 |
| ii | 2 | xv | 15 |
| iii | 3 | xx | 20 |
| iv | 4 | xxx | 30 |
| v | 5 | L | 50 |
| vi | 6 | C | 100 |
| vii | 7 | D | 500 |
| viii | 8 | M | 1000 |

*Practice Problems*

Change to Roman numerals

1.　2 _____

2.　5 _____

3.　7 _____

4.　12 _____

5.　31 _____

Change to Arabic numerals

6.　iii _____

7.　iv _____

8.　xxv _____

9.　xvi _____

10.　viii _____

# Multiplication of Whole Numbers

The multiplication table below is provided for review. Study the table and test yourself. You should achieve 100% without referring to the table.

### Multiplication Table

| 1  | 2  | 3  | 4  | 5  | 6  | 7  | 8  | 9   | 10  | 11  | 12  |
|----|----|----|----|----|----|----|----|-----|-----|-----|-----|
| 2  | 4  | 6  | 8  | 10 | 12 | 14 | 16 | 18  | 20  | 22  | 24  |
| 3  | 6  | 9  | 12 | 15 | 18 | 21 | 24 | 27  | 30  | 33  | 36  |
| 4  | 8  | 12 | 16 | 20 | 24 | 28 | 32 | 36  | 40  | 44  | 48  |
| 5  | 10 | 15 | 20 | 25 | 30 | 35 | 40 | 45  | 50  | 55  | 60  |
| 6  | 12 | 18 | 24 | 30 | 36 | 42 | 48 | 54  | 60  | 66  | 72  |
| 7  | 14 | 21 | 28 | 35 | 42 | 49 | 56 | 63  | 70  | 77  | 84  |
| 8  | 16 | 24 | 32 | 40 | 48 | 56 | 64 | 72  | 80  | 88  | 96  |
| 9  | 18 | 27 | 36 | 45 | 54 | 63 | 72 | 81  | 90  | 99  | 108 |
| 10 | 20 | 30 | 40 | 50 | 60 | 70 | 80 | 90  | 100 | 110 | 120 |
| 11 | 12 | 33 | 44 | 55 | 66 | 77 | 88 | 99  | 110 | 121 | 132 |
| 12 | 24 | 36 | 48 | 60 | 72 | 84 | 96 | 108 | 120 | 132 | 144 |

To multiply any two numbers from 1-12, find a number in the vertical column then find a number in the horizontal column. Read across until the vertical and horizontal columns intersect. Example: 6 x 8 = 48

Test yourself:

1. 2 x 7 =

2. 3 x 9 =

3. 4 x 8 =

4. 5 x 9 =

5. 6 x 7 =

6. 7 x 8 =

7. 8 x 6 =

8. 8 x 5 =

9. 9 x 4 =

10. 7 x 5 =

11. 8 x 5 =

12. 6 x 12 =

13. 9 x 9 =

14. 9 x 7 =

15. 7 x 12 =

# Decimals

Medications are frequently prescribed in decimals. This section will provide a review of addition, subtraction, multiplication and division of decimals, and the relative value of decimals.

## Addition of Decimals

To add the decimals, place the decimal points exactly under one another. If you want to add 0.5, 2.25 and 6.0, place the numbers as below.

$$
\begin{array}{r}
0.5 \\
2.25 \\
\underline{6.00} \\
8.75
\end{array}
$$

Place the decimal point in the answer, directly under the aligned decimal points.

**Note:** *Line up the decimal points before adding. Add from right to left. To add or subtract decimals, add zeros to avoid confusion. Example: 2.4 + .5  Add zero before the decimal point.  2.4 + 0.5*

*Practice Problems*

**Line up and add**

11.  2.3 + 0.05

12.  5.2 + 0.5

13.  0.06 + 0.4

14.  3.1 + 0.234

15.  0.5 + 3.24 + 6

16.  88.818 + 45.123

17.  17.522 + 74.561

18.  7.44 + 3.04 + 11.31

19.  6.42 + 9.55 + 13.2

20.  0.8 + 0.5

21.  10.56 + 356.4

22.  3.27 + 0.06 + 2

# Subtraction of Decimals

Place the decimals to be subtracted directly under the decimal of the larger number. If you subtract 3.1 from 5.2, the numbers should be placed as below.

```
5.2
3.1
```

Place the decimal point in the answer directly under the aligned decimal points.

```
 5.2
-3.1
─────
 2.1
```

*Practice Problems*

**Subtract**

23. 6.2 – 4.1

24. 4.3 – 2.1

25. 6 – 2.6

26. 16.84 – 1.32

27. 13.6 – 7

28. 83.664 – 25.888

29. 48.638 – 37.796

30. 266.44 – 0.56

31. 0.8100 – 0.6701

32. 98.6 – 66.50

33. 7.066 – 0.100

34. 21.78 – 19.88

# Multiplication of Decimals

Multiply decimals using the same method as whole numbers.

```
     6.3
   x 4.3
   ─────
    18 9

    252
   ─────
   27.09
```

After multiplying, count off the number of decimal places to the right of the decimal. Then count that total and place it right to left in the product.

```
     6.3      one place
   x 4.3      one place
   ─────
    18 9

    252
   ─────
   27.0 9     two places
```

To multiply by 10, 100 or 1000 simply move the decimal point to the right as many places as there are zeros in the multiplier.

| | |
|---|---|
| 0.613 x 10 | There is one zero in the multiplier |
| 0 6.13 | Decimal is moved one place to the right |
| | |
| 0.613 x 100 | There are two zeros in the multiplier |
| 61.3 | Decimal is moved two places to the right |
| | |
| 0.613 x 1000 | There are three zeros in the multiplier |
| 613. | Decimal is moved three places to the right |

*Practice Problems*

## Multtiply

35. $4.8 \times 2.1$

36. $63.8 \times 0.9$

37. $7 \times 4.97$

38. $0.007 \times 10$

39. $35.1 \times 1000$

40. $8.5 \times 0.96$

41. $7.54 \times 5.2$

42. $0.5 \times 100$

43. $90.1 \times 88$

44. $36.8 \times 70.1$

45. $54.1 \times 21$

46. $0.03 \times 1.2$

# Division of Decimals

To divide a decimal by a whole number, place the decimal point in the quotient, directly above the decimal point in the dividend.

$$\text{Divisor} \overline{)\,\text{Dividend}}^{\text{Quotient}}$$

$$5 \overline{)\,5.25}^{1.05}$$

To divide by 10, 100 or 1000
Move the decimal point the same number of places to the left as there are zeros in the divisor.

    0.8/10  =      0.08
    0.8/100 =       .008
    0.8/1000 =      .0008

To divide a decimal by a decimal, use a caret to "move" the decimal point.

Example 1    1.    $0.8 \overline{)\,2.864}$

             2.    $0.8 \overline{)\,2.864}$

        *move one place*          *move one place*

             3.         $8. \overline{)\,28.64}^{3.58}$

Example 2    1.    $0.12 \overline{)\,.04416}$

             2.    $0.12 \overline{)\,.04416}$

   *move two places*          *move two places*

             3.    $12. \overline{)\,04.416}^{.368}$

**Divide**

47. 3.936 ÷ 32.8

48. 63.9 ÷ 0.9

49. 0.098 ÷ 0.7

50. 0.007 ÷ 10

51. 35.1 ÷ 1000

52. 3 ÷ 25

53. 0.30 ÷ 20

54. 4 ÷ 25

55. 0.01 ÷ 0.02

56. 76.53 ÷ 10

57. 10.8 ÷ 0.02

58. 15.06 ÷ 6

59. 158.4 ÷ 48

60. 650.80 ÷ 0.70

# Relative Value of Decimal Fractions

Decimal fractions are referred to as decimals. 0.2 is a decimal fraction or decimal. $0.2(\text{decimal}) = \frac{2}{10}$ (fraction)

Remember the numbers to the right of the decimals have a value less than 1. Note the following chart.

**Decimal Point**

Thousands    Hundreds    Tens    Ones    .    .1     .01     .001     .0001

**Note:** *On the left side of the chart the numbers rise in value from one to tens to hundreds etc. On the right side of the chart the decimal numbers have a value of less than one.*

    Example:   10.1 is greater than 9
                 .1 is greater than .01

The numbers to the right of the decimal point indicate tenths, hundredths, and thousandths, in that order.

The decimal fraction which has the larger number representing the tenths has the greater value. 0.4 has a greater value than 0.2

If in decimal fractions the numbers representing the tenths are identical then the number representing the hundreths will determine the value. The largest number in the hundredths will have the greatest value.

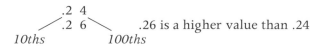

The tenths are the same .2 and .2. The next numbers, 4 and 6 are in the hundredths column.
6 is higher than 4

**Which is the greater value?**

61. a  0.4          b  0.35          c  0.5

62. a  0.24          b  0.25          c  0.26

63. a  0.125          b  0.1          c  0.05

64. a  0.6          b  0.16          c  0.06

65. If you have a tablet with a strength of 0.2 and you need to give 0.5, you will need:
    a  one tablet     b  less than 1 tablet     c  more than 1 tablet

**Which number has the greatest value?**

66. a  11.04          b  10.19          c  12.01

67. a  6.14          b  4.95          c  3.54

68. a  3.55          b  2.95          c  3.8

**Reading Decimal Fractions**

To read decimals fractions, read the number to the right of the decimal and use the name that applies to that place value of the last figure.

Example:
0.356          = Three hundred fifty-six thousandths.
0.3056          = Three thousand fifty-six ten thousandths
0.30056          = Thirty thousand fifty-six hundred thousandths

**Read the following out loud.**

70.  0.07

71.  0.082

72.  0.0016

73.  0.0005

**Express the following as a decimal.**

74.  Forty-six hundredths

75.  Two thousandths

76.  Four hundredths

77.  Thirty-two and one tenth

# Fractions

Many drug preparations are prescribed and prepared in fractions. You will need to have an understanding of fractions and be able to add, subtract, multiply and divide fractions.

numerator    -    number on top    - $\dfrac{1}{2}$
denominator  -    number on bottom -

A fraction is a portion of a whole and indicates division of that whole.

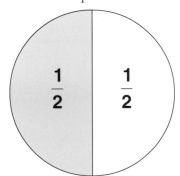
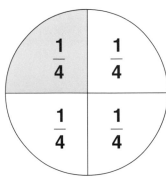
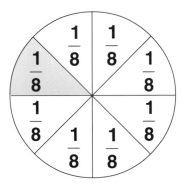

$\dfrac{1}{2}$ is larger than $\dfrac{1}{4}$ or $\dfrac{1}{8}$     $\dfrac{1}{2}$ is a larger portion of the whole than is     $\dfrac{1}{4}$ or $\dfrac{1}{8}$

### The numerator of a fraction

The numerator tells you how many of the equal parts you have. In $\dfrac{3}{5}$ , the numerator 3 tells you there are 3 equal parts that are each worth $\dfrac{1}{5}$

If the numerator is equal to the denominator, the fraction is equal to 1

$\dfrac{3}{3} = 1$        $\dfrac{4}{4} = 1$

If the numerator is greater than the denominator, the fraction is equal to more than one.

Example    $\dfrac{5}{4}$

Divide the denominator into the numerator        $\dfrac{5}{4} = 1\dfrac{1}{4}$

### The denominator of a fraction

The denominator of a fraction tells you the number of equal parts into which a whole has been divided. In $\frac{1}{8}$ the eight tells you a whole has been divided into 8 equal parts.

## Terminology:

Proper fraction- numerator is less than denominator

Improper fraction - numerator is greater than the denominator

Mixed fraction - whole number and fraction combined.

Common fraction - refers to proper fractions, improper fraction and mixed numbers.

# Addition of Fractions

**To add fractions with like denominators:**

Add the numerators.  The denominators stay the same.

Example:  $\dfrac{2}{8} + \dfrac{3}{8} = \dfrac{5}{8}$

Numerators $2 + 3 = 5$
The denominators (8 ) do not change.

**To add fractions with unlike denominators, find a common denominator.**

The easiest way to find a common denominator is to multiply the denominators.
In the addition problem of: $\dfrac{1}{4} + \dfrac{3}{5}$

4 and 5 are the denominators.

To find the common denominator multiply 4 x 5.
$4x5 = 20$      20 is the common denominator.

Divide the common denominator, 20, by the denominator of each fraction

$$4\overline{)20} = 5 \qquad 5\overline{)20} = 4$$

Multiply the result with the numerators      $5 \times 1 = 5$
$4 \times 3 = 12$

$$\dfrac{1}{4} + \dfrac{3}{5} =$$

$$\dfrac{5}{20} + \dfrac{12}{20}$$

Add:  $\dfrac{5}{20} + \dfrac{12}{20} = \dfrac{17}{20}$

**To add fractions with a mixed number, follow these steps:**

1. Change the mixed number to an improper fraction.

   To add $\frac{1}{3}$ and $2\frac{3}{8}$ and $\frac{2}{3}$    Change $2\frac{3}{8}$ to $\frac{19}{8}$ by multiplying $2 \times 8$ than adding the numerator 3 to 16.  The 19 is now the numerator and 8 is the denominator.

   Example :    $2\frac{3}{8} = \frac{8 \times 2 + 3}{8} = \frac{19}{8}$

   The mixed number $2\frac{3}{8}$ is now an improper fraction $\frac{19}{8}$

   Example :    $\frac{1}{3} + 2\frac{3}{8} + \frac{2}{3} = \frac{1}{3} + \frac{19}{8} + \frac{2}{3}$

2. Find a common denominator.

   Find the lowest common number that the bottom numbers can be divided into evenly. The common denominator can be found by multiplying 3 x 8.

   Example:    $3 \times 8 = 24$

   24 is the lowest common number that the bottom numbers can be divided into evenly.

3. Change unlike fractions to like fractions.

   Change the fractions into equivalent fractions by using the common denominator.

   Example :    $\frac{1}{3} + \frac{19}{8} + \frac{2}{3} = \frac{8}{24} + \frac{57}{24} + \frac{16}{24}$

   Example :    $\frac{1}{3} = \frac{8}{24}$        $\frac{19}{8} = \frac{57}{24}$        $\frac{2}{3} = \frac{16}{24}$

4. Add the numerators

   Example:    $\frac{8}{24} + \frac{57}{24} + \frac{16}{24} = \frac{81}{24} = 3\frac{9}{24}$ or $3\frac{3}{8}$

**Add the fractions**

78. $\dfrac{5}{11} + \dfrac{9}{11} + \dfrac{13}{11}$

79. $6\dfrac{1}{6} + 9\dfrac{3}{8}$

80. $\dfrac{5}{20} + \dfrac{8}{20} + \dfrac{13}{20}$

81. $2\dfrac{1}{4} + 3\dfrac{1}{8}$

82. $\dfrac{1}{4} + 2\dfrac{5}{8}$

83. $\dfrac{3}{4} + \dfrac{2}{5}$

84. $\dfrac{1}{2} + \dfrac{2}{5}$

85. $\dfrac{1}{2} + \dfrac{1}{3}$

86. $\dfrac{3}{10} + \dfrac{1}{8}$

87. $\dfrac{3}{4} + \dfrac{4}{5}$

88. $\dfrac{2}{5} + \dfrac{2}{5}$

89. $2\dfrac{1}{3} + 4\dfrac{1}{6}$

90. $\dfrac{3}{5} + \dfrac{2}{3}$

91. $8\dfrac{2}{5} + 9\dfrac{9}{10} + 14\dfrac{7}{10}$

92. $9\dfrac{5}{8} + 6\dfrac{1}{6}$

# Subtraction of Fractions

To subtract fractions with like denominators, subtract the numerators.

$$\frac{5}{6} - \frac{2}{6} = \frac{3}{6}$$

To subtract fractions with unlike denominators, find a common denominator.

$\frac{5}{6} - \frac{2}{5}$      $\frac{5}{6}$ becomes $\frac{25}{30}$      $\frac{2}{5}$ becomes $\frac{12}{30}$

$$\frac{25}{30} - \frac{12}{30} = \frac{13}{30}$$

To subtract fractions with a mixed number, follow these steps

1. Change the mixed number to an improper fraction

   To subtract $\frac{1}{3}$ from $2\frac{1}{4}$ change $2\frac{1}{4}$ to $\frac{9}{4}$

   Now you have $\frac{9}{4} - \frac{1}{3}$

2. Find a common denominator.
   The common denominator for 4 and 3 is 12.

3. Change the unlike fractions to like fractions.

   $\frac{9}{4}$ becomes $\frac{27}{12}$      $\frac{1}{3}$ becomes $\frac{4}{12}$

   Now you have $\frac{27}{12} - \frac{4}{12}$

4. Subtract the numerators

   $\frac{27}{12} - \frac{4}{12} = \frac{23}{12}$      Reduced $\frac{23}{12} = 1\frac{11}{12}$

Subtract the fractions

93. $\dfrac{3}{5} - \dfrac{1}{6}$

94. $\dfrac{8}{9} - \dfrac{4}{9}$

95. $\dfrac{5}{7} - \dfrac{2}{7}$

96. $\dfrac{3}{4} - \dfrac{2}{9}$

97. $2\dfrac{1}{4} - \dfrac{2}{3}$

98. $\dfrac{7}{8} - \dfrac{3}{8}$

99. $\dfrac{5}{6} - \dfrac{4}{6}$

100. $\dfrac{5}{6} - \dfrac{3}{8}$

101. $\dfrac{2}{3} - \dfrac{1}{2}$

102. $\dfrac{5}{6} - \dfrac{2}{3}$

103. $1\dfrac{1}{10} - \dfrac{3}{5}$

104. $\dfrac{4}{5} - \dfrac{1}{2}$

105. $2\dfrac{7}{8} - \dfrac{3}{4}$

106. $\dfrac{7}{8} - \dfrac{2}{3}$

107. $7 - 1\dfrac{3}{4}$

# Multiplication of Fractions

To multiply fractions, you merely multiply the numerators by each other and multiply the denominators by each other.

Multiply the numerators of fractions to get the new numerator.

Multiply the denominators of fractions to get the new denominator.

$$\frac{3}{4} \times \frac{1}{3} = \frac{3}{12} \qquad \text{Reduced} \quad \frac{3}{12} = \frac{1}{4}$$

A short cut method of multiplying fractions involves cancellation before multiplying.

$$\frac{\cancel{3}}{4} \times \frac{1}{\cancel{3}} = \frac{1}{4}$$

To multiply a fraction that involves a mixed number, change the mixed number to an improper fraction.

$$2\frac{1}{4} \times \frac{1}{2} = \frac{9}{4} \times \frac{1}{2} \qquad\qquad \frac{9}{4} \times \frac{1}{2} = \frac{9}{8}$$

# Division of Fractions

To divide fractions follow these steps:

1.  Invert the number by which you are dividing.

$$\frac{4}{5} \div \frac{5}{9} \quad \text{Invert} \quad \frac{5}{9} \quad \text{to} \quad \frac{9}{5}$$

2.  Multiply the fractions to get the answer.

$$\frac{4}{5} \times \frac{9}{5} = \frac{36}{25} \qquad \text{Reduced} \frac{36}{25} = 1\frac{11}{25}$$

To divide a fraction that involves a mixed number, change the mixed number to an improper fraction, invert, than multiply.

$$\frac{1}{2} \div 1\frac{3}{5} \quad \text{change} \quad 1\frac{3}{5} \text{ to } \frac{8}{5} \qquad \frac{1}{2} \div \frac{8}{5}$$

$$\text{Invert} \quad \frac{8}{5} \text{ to } \frac{5}{8}$$

$$\text{Multiply} \quad \frac{1}{2} \times \frac{5}{8} = \frac{5}{16}$$

**Multiply and Divide the fractions**

108. $\dfrac{5}{9} \times \dfrac{2}{7}$

109. $\dfrac{3}{4} \times \dfrac{6}{7}$

110. $2\dfrac{3}{4} \times \dfrac{1}{3}$

111. $3\dfrac{1}{2} \times \dfrac{3}{16}$

112. $\dfrac{4}{5} \times 2\dfrac{1}{2}$

113. $\dfrac{2}{3} \times \dfrac{5}{8}$

114. $\dfrac{7}{8} \times \dfrac{2}{3}$

115. $\dfrac{1}{9} \times \dfrac{2}{3}$

116. $\dfrac{1}{2} \times \dfrac{3}{7}$

117. $2\dfrac{3}{5} \times 1\dfrac{1}{3}$

118. $\dfrac{3}{10} \times \dfrac{1}{12}$

119. $\dfrac{5}{8} \times 1\dfrac{1}{6}$

120. $\dfrac{12}{25} \times \dfrac{3}{5}$

121. $\dfrac{1}{100} \times 3$

122. $\dfrac{1}{5} \times \dfrac{1}{3}$

123. $\dfrac{3}{8} \div \dfrac{2}{3}$

124. $\dfrac{1}{100} \div \dfrac{1}{4}$

125. $\dfrac{6}{7} \div \dfrac{1}{3}$

126. $\dfrac{5}{8} \div \dfrac{7}{12}$

127. $\dfrac{6}{13} \div \dfrac{2}{3}$

128. $\dfrac{3}{8} \div \dfrac{7}{20}$

129. $3\dfrac{5}{6} \div \dfrac{3}{7}$

130. $\dfrac{1}{2} \div \dfrac{5}{8}$

131. $\dfrac{3}{4} \div 3$

132. $\dfrac{1}{60} \div \dfrac{1}{2}$

133. $2\dfrac{1}{2} \div \dfrac{3}{4}$

134. $\dfrac{1}{150} \div \dfrac{1}{50}$

135. $\dfrac{2}{5} \div \dfrac{5}{8}$

136. $4 \div 2\dfrac{1}{8}$

137. $2 \div \dfrac{1}{5}$

# Ratios

A ratio is composed of two numbers separated by a colon.  These two numbers are related to each other.

> Example:   1 : 100
>> There is a relationship between the 1 and 100.  This ratio of 1:100 could represent
>> 1 tablet :  100 mg  (One tablet contains 100 mg.)

> Example:   1: 50
>> This ratio could represent 1 tab: 50 mg. (1 tablet contains 50 mg)

The ratio of how many mg in each tablet is stated on the drug label.

Two ratios separated by an equal (=) sign indicates a proportion.

> Example:   1: 50  =  2 : 100
>> If one tablet contains 50 mg, then 2 tablets would contain 100 mg.

For more information on ratios see Chapter 2.


## Solve for X

If  3 numbers of two ratios are known, the 4th number can be found.

> Example:   1: 50   =  X : 100

>> Multiply     50 x X

>> Multiply     1 x 100

>> 50 X = 100

> Example :   $\dfrac{1}{50} = \dfrac{X}{100}$

To solve for X using a common fraction, set the problem up as follows

Cross Multiply   $\dfrac{1}{50} \times \dfrac{X}{100}$

$$50 X = 100$$

$$X = \dfrac{100}{50}$$

$$X = 2$$

# Ratios *cont.*

Make sure when setting up the proportion that the ratios are written in the same sequence of measurement units.

Example  $\dfrac{10 \text{ mg}}{1 \text{ mL}} = \dfrac{5 \text{ mg}}{X \text{ mL}}$

Like units on the top are the same (mg)
Like units on the bottom are the same (mL)

$$\dfrac{10 \text{ mg}}{1 \text{ mL}} \diagup\!\!\!\!\diagdown \dfrac{5 \text{ mg}}{X \text{ mL}}$$

$$10 \text{ X} = 5$$

$$X = 0.5 \text{ mL}$$

*Practice Problems*

**Solve for X**

138.  $\dfrac{5}{3} = \dfrac{25}{X}$     X=

139.  $\dfrac{1}{200} = \dfrac{X}{5000}$     X=

140.  $\dfrac{8}{39} = \dfrac{16}{X}$     X=

141.  $\dfrac{5}{20} = \dfrac{X}{40}$     X=

142.  $\dfrac{9}{X} = \dfrac{5}{300}$     X=

143.  $\dfrac{250}{1} = \dfrac{750}{X}$     X=

144.  $\dfrac{6}{24} = \dfrac{0.75}{X}$     X=

# Percent

Percent (%) means parts per hundred. Percent can be used to express the number of grams of drug per 100 mL of solvent.

Example: 100 mL of 2 % solution will contain 2 grams of drug.
To determine the grams, multiply 100 mL x 2 %.
Change 2 % to a decimal by dividing by 100
2 divided by 100 = .02

100 x .02 = 2

Example: 100 mL of 1 % solution will contain 1 gram of drug.
To determine the gram, multiply 100 x .01

100 x .01 = 1

How many grams of drug will 50 mL of a 10 % solution contain? _____

Answer: 5 grams

How many grams of drug will 200 mL of a 10% solution contain? _____

Answer: 20 grams

# Equivalents of Decimals, Fractions, Ratios and Percents

Drug dosages may be expressed as decimals, fractions, ratios and percents. These measures can be expressed as equivalents of each other.

Example:

$\frac{1}{5}$    0.2 grams    ½ gram    1:5    20 %

decimal    fraction    ratio    percent

The above decimal, fraction, ratio and percents are equivalents.

### Change a Decimal to a Common Fraction

To change a decimal to a common fraction, change the decimal number to a whole number and place it in the numerator.
For the denominator, place a 1 plus as many spaces as are to the right of the decimal point.
Reduce to lowest terms.

Example: Decimal 0.20    Convert 0.20 to a fraction.

$\frac{20}{100} = \frac{1}{5}$    Nominator 20 / Denominator 100

## Change a Fraction to a Decimal

To convert a fraction to a decimal, divide the numerator by the denominator.

Example:   Convert $\dfrac{1}{3}$ to a decimal.

$$\dfrac{1}{3} = 1 \div 3 \qquad 1 \div 3 = 0.33$$

## Change a Fraction to a Ratio
To change a fraction to a ratio, simply change the position of the numbers.

Example:

$$\dfrac{1}{5} \;=\; 1:5$$

## Change a Decimal, Ratio or Common Fraction to a Percent
To change to percent, multiply by 100.
Percent is obtained by multiplying by 100 and adding the % sign.

Example:
            Decimal 0.5 x 100 =  50 %

        Ratio 1 : 2   or Fraction   $\frac{1}{2}$ x $^{100}/_1$  =  50 %

### *Practice Problems*

Find the ratio, common fraction and percent from these decimals.

|      | Decimal | Ratio | Common Fraction | Percent |
|------|---------|-------|-----------------|---------|
| 145. | 0.5     | a_____ | b _____       | c _____ |
| 146. | 0.1     | a_____ | b _____       | c _____ |
| 147. | 0.9     | a_____ | b _____       | c _____ |

Find the decimals, ratio and common fractions from these percents.

|      | Percents | Ratio | Common Fraction | Decimal |
|------|----------|-------|-----------------|---------|
| 148. | 25 %     | a_____ | b _____       | c _____ |
| 149. | 5%       | a_____ | b _____       | c _____ |
| 150. | 4 %      | a_____ | b _____       | c _____ |

# Answer Key for Math Review

| | | | | | | | |
|---|---|---|---|---|---|---|---|
| 1 | ii | 44. | 2579.68 | 81. | $5\frac{3}{8}$ | 96. | $\frac{19}{36}$ |
| 2 | v | 45. | 1136.1 | | | | |
| 3 | vii | 46. | 0.036 | | | | |
| 4 | xii | 47. | 0.12 | 82. | $2\frac{7}{8}$ | 97. | $1\frac{7}{12}$ |
| 5 | xxxi | 48. | 71 | | | | |
| 6 | 3 | 49. | 0.14 | | | | |
| 7 | 4 | 50. | 0.0007 | 83. | $1\frac{3}{20}$ | 98. | $\frac{1}{2}$ |
| 8 | 25 | 51 | 0.0351 | | | | |
| 9 | 16 | 52. | 0.12 | | | | |
| 10 | 8 | 53. | 0.015 | 84. | $\frac{9}{10}$ | 99. | $\frac{1}{6}$ |
| 11 | 2.35 | 54. | 0.16 | | | | |
| 12 | 5.7 | 55. | 0.5 | | | | |
| 13 | 0.46 | 56. | 7.653 | 85. | $\frac{5}{6}$ | 100. | $\frac{11}{24}$ |
| 14 | 3.334 | 57. | 540 | | | | |
| 15 | 9.74 | 58. | 2.51 | | | | |
| 16. | 133.941 | 59. | 3.3 | 86. | $\frac{17}{40}$ | 101. | $\frac{1}{6}$ |
| 17. | 92.083 | 60. | 929.7 | | | | |
| 18. | 21.79 | 61. | c 0.5 | | | | |
| 19. | 29.17 | 62 | c 0.26 | 87. | $1\frac{11}{20}$ | 102. | $\frac{1}{6}$ |
| 20. | 1.3 | 63. | a 0.125 | | | | |
| 21. | 366.96 | 64. | a 0.6 | | | | |
| 22. | 5.33 | 65. | c more than 1 | 88. | $\frac{4}{5}$ | 103. | $\frac{1}{2}$ |
| 23. | 2.1 | | tablet | | | | |
| 24. | 2.2 | 66. | c 12.01 | | | | |
| 25. | 3.4 | 67. | a 6.14 | 89. | $6\frac{1}{2}$ | 104. | $\frac{3}{10}$ |
| 26. | 15.52 | 68. | c 3.8 | | | | |
| 27. | 6.6 | 69. | b 7.5 | | | | |
| 28. | 57.776 | 70. | Seven hundredths | 90. | $1\frac{4}{15}$ | 105. | $2\frac{1}{8}$ |
| 29. | 10.842 | 71. | Eighty-two | | | | |
| 30. | 265.88 | | thousandths | | | | |
| 31. | 0.1399 | 72. | Sixteen ten | 91. | 33 | 106. | $\frac{5}{24}$ |
| 32. | 32.1 | | thousandths | | | | |
| 33. | 6.966 | 73. | Five ten thou | 92. | $15\frac{19}{24}$ | | |
| 34. | 1.9 | | sandths | | | 107. | $5\frac{1}{4}$ |
| 35. | 10.08 | 74. | 0.46 | | | | |
| 36. | 57.42 | 75. | 0.002 | 93. | $\frac{13}{30}$ | | |
| 37. | 34.79 | 76. | 0.04 | | | 108. | $\frac{10}{63}$ |
| 38. | 0.07 | 77. | 32.1 | | | | |
| 39. | 35,100 | | | 94. | $\frac{4}{9}$ | | |
| 40. | 8.16 | | | | | 109. | $\frac{9}{14}$ |
| 41. | 39.208 | 78. | $2\frac{5}{11}$ | | | | |
| 42. | 50 | | | 95. | $\frac{3}{7}$ | | |
| 43. | 7928.8 | 79. | $15\frac{13}{24}$ | | | | |
| | | 80. | $1\frac{3}{10}$ | | | | |

# Answer Key for Math Review *cont.*

110. $\dfrac{11}{12}$

111. $\dfrac{21}{32}$

112. $\dfrac{20}{10}$ or 2

113. $\dfrac{5}{12}$

114. $\dfrac{7}{12}$

115. $\dfrac{2}{27}$

116. $\dfrac{3}{14}$

117. $3\dfrac{7}{15}$

118. $\dfrac{1}{40}$

119. $\dfrac{35}{48}$

120. $\dfrac{36}{125}$

121. $\dfrac{3}{100}$

122. $\dfrac{1}{15}$

123. $\dfrac{9}{16}$

124. $\dfrac{1}{25}$

125. $2\dfrac{4}{7}$

126. $1\dfrac{1}{14}$

127. $\dfrac{9}{13}$

128. $1\dfrac{1}{14}$

129. $8\dfrac{17}{18}$

130. $\dfrac{4}{5}$

131. $\dfrac{1}{4}$

132. $\dfrac{1}{30}$

133. $3\dfrac{1}{3}$

134. $\dfrac{1}{3}$

135. $\dfrac{16}{25}$

136. $1\dfrac{15}{17}$

137. 10

138. 15

139. 25

140  78

141. 10

142. 540

143. 3

144. 3

| Decimal | Ratio | Common Fraction | Percent |
|---|---|---|---|
| 145. 0.5 | a 1: 2 | b $\dfrac{1}{2}$ | c 50 % |
| 146. 0.1 | a 1: 10 | b $\dfrac{1}{10}$ | c 10 % |
| 147. 0.9 | a 9: 10 | b $\dfrac{9}{10}$ | c 90 % |

| Percent | Ratio | Common Fraction | Decimal |
|---|---|---|---|
| 148. 25 % | a 1: 4 | b $\dfrac{1}{4}$ | c 0.25 |
| 149. 5 % | a 1: 20 | b $\dfrac{1}{20}$ | c 0.05 |
| 150. 4 % | a 1: 25 | b $\dfrac{1}{25}$ | c 0.04 |

# INDEX

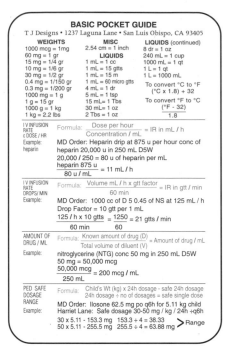

### BASIC POCKET GUIDE
T J Designs • 1237 Laguna Lane • San Luis Obispo, CA 93405

| WEIGHTS | MISC | LIQUIDS (continued) |
|---|---|---|
| 1000 mcg = 1mg | 2.54 cm = 1 inch | 8 dr = 1 oz |
| 60 mg = 1 gr | **LIQUIDS** | 240 mL = 1 cup |
| 15 mg = 1/4 gr | 1 mL = 1 cc | 1000 mL = 1 qt |
| 10 mg = 1/6 gr | 1 mL = 15 gtts | 1 L = 1 qt |
| 30 mg = 1/2 gr | 1 mL = 15 m | 1 L = 1000 mL |
| 0.4 mg = 1/150 gr | 1 mL = 60 micro gtts | To convert °C to °F |
| 0.3 mg = 1/200 gr | 4 mL = 1 dr | (°C x 1.8) + 32 |
| 1000 mg = 1 g | 5 mL = 1 tsp | To convert °F to °C |
| 1 g = 15 gr | 15 mL = 1 Tbs | (°F - 32) |
| 1000 g = 1 kg | 30 mL = 1 oz | ————— |
| 1 kg = 2.2 lbs | 2 Tbs = 1 oz | 1.8 |

**I V INFUSION RATE c DOSE / HR** — Formula: $\dfrac{\text{Dose per hour}}{\text{Concentration / mL}} = \text{IR in mL / h}$

Example: heparin — MD Order: Heparin drip at 875 u per hour conc of heparin 20,000 u in 250 mL D5W

20,000 / 250 = 80 u of heparin per mL

$\dfrac{\text{heparin 875 u}}{80 \text{ u / mL}} = 11 \text{ mL / h}$

**I V INFUSION RATE DROPS/ MIN** — Formula: $\dfrac{\text{Volume mL / h x gtt factor}}{60 \text{ min}} = \text{IR in gtt / min}$

Example: MD Order: 1000 cc of D 5 0.45 of NS at 125 mL / h
Drop Factor = 10 gtt per 1 mL

$\dfrac{125 / h \times 10 \text{ gtts}}{60 \text{ min}} = \dfrac{1250}{60} = 21 \text{ gtts / min}$

**AMOUNT OF DRUG / ML** — Formula: $\dfrac{\text{Known amount of drug (D)}}{\text{Total volume of diluent (V)}} = \text{Amount of drug / mL}$

Example: nitroglycerine (NTG) conc 50 mg in 250 mL D5W
50 mg = 50,000 mcg

$\dfrac{50,000 \text{ mcg}}{250 \text{ mL}} = 200 \text{ mcg / mL}$

**PED SAFE DOSAGE RANGE** — Formula: $\dfrac{\text{Child's Wt (kg) x 24h dosage - safe 24h dosage}}{24\text{h dosage} \div \text{no of dosages}} = \text{safe single dose}$

Example: MD Order: Ilosone 62.5 mg po q6h for 5.11 kg child
Harriet Lane: Safe dosage 30-50 mg / kg / 24h ÷q6h

30 x 5.11 - 153.3 mg   153.3 ÷ 4 = 38.33  } Range
50 x 5.11 - 255.5 mg   255.5 ÷ 4 = 63.88 mg

### Pocket Guide A

### CRITICAL CARE POCKET GUIDE
T J Designs • 1237 Laguna Lane • San Luis Obispo, CA 93405

**DOSE/MIN** — Formula: $\dfrac{\text{Conc per mL x infusion rate}}{60 \text{ min}} = \text{Dose / min}$

Example nitro-glycerine — MD Order: Titrate nitroglycerine (NTG) drip for relief of chest pains. NTG conc is 50 in 250 of D5W nitroglycerine 200 mcg per mL

$\dfrac{\text{NTG 200 mcg / mL x 3 mL / h}}{60 \text{ min}} = 10 \text{ mcg / min}$

**IR IN mL / h c DOSE / MIN** — Formula: $\dfrac{\text{Desired dose / min x 60 mL / h}}{\text{Conc. / mL}} = \text{IR mL / h}$

Example: MD Orders to start NTG at 5 mcg / min titrate until chest pain is relieved.

$\dfrac{5 \text{ mcg x 60 mL / h}}{200 \text{ mcg / mL}} = \dfrac{300}{200} = 2 \text{ mL / h}$

**CONC. FX. FOR MCG / KG / MIN** — Formula: $\dfrac{\dfrac{\text{Mcg / mL}}{\text{Weight (kg)}}}{60 \text{ min}} = \text{Concentration Factor}$

Example dopamine — Dopamine Conc 400 mg / 250 of D5W or 1600 mcg / mL Patient's weight is 123 lbs / 2.2 = 56 kg

$\dfrac{1600 \text{ mcg / mL}}{56 \text{ kg}} = 28.57 \quad \dfrac{28.57}{60 \text{ min}} = \boxed{0.476 \text{ SAVE}} \text{ Conc Fx}$

**MCG / KG / MIN** — Formula: Conc. Factor x mL / h = mcg / kg / min

Example dopamine — Dopamine Conc Fx is 0.476 and the infusion rate is15 mL / h How many mcg / kg is this per min?
0.476 (Conc Fx) x 15 mL / h = 7 mcg / kg / min

**IR c DOSE MCG / KG / MIN** — Formula: $\dfrac{\text{mcg / kg / min}}{\text{Conc Fx}} = \text{Infusion Rate}$

Example dopamine — MD Order: Give 3 mcg / kg / min of dopamine The conc Fx is 0.476 (see above)

$\dfrac{3 \text{ mcg / kg / min}}{0.476 \text{ (Conc Fx)}} = 6 \text{ mL / h}$

### Pocket Guide B

| Drug (Double Conc.) | Maintenance | Maximum | Concentration | Con./ml |
|---|---|---|---|---|
| **DRUGS ORDERED IN MG/MIN** | | | | |
| bretylium (Bretylol) | 1-2 mg/min | 2 mg/min | 2 Gm/250 mL D5W | 8 mg/mL |
| lidocaine (Xylocaine) | 1-4 mg/min | 4 mg/min | 2 Gm/250 mL D5W | 8 mg/mL |
| procainamide (Pronestyl) | 2-6 mg/min | 2-6 mg/min | 2 Gm/250 mL D5W | 8 mg/mL |
| **DRUGS ORDERED IN MCG/MIN** | | | | |
| epinephrine (Adrenaline) | 1-4 mcg/min | 4 mcg/min | 2 mg/250 mL D5W | 8 mcg/mL |
| isoproterenol (Isuprel) | 0.5-5 mcg/min | 30 mcg/min | 2 mg/250 mL D5W | 8 mcg/mL |
| nitroglycerin (Tridil) | 5-400 mcg/min | 400 mcg/min | 50 mg/250 mL D5W | 200 mcg/mL |
| norepinephrine (Levophed) | 2-4 mcg/min | 47 mcg/min | 4 mg/250 mL D5W | 16 mcg/mL |
| phenylephrine (Neo-Synephrine) | 40-60 mcg/min | 180 mcg/min | 10 mg/250 mL D5WL | 40 mcg/mL |
| **DRUGS ORDERED IN UNITS/MIN** | | | | |
| vasopressin (Pitressin) | 0.1-0.9 u/min | 0.9 u/min | 150 u/150 mL D5W | 1 u/mL |
| **DRUGS ORDERED IN MCG/KG/MIN** | | | | |
| amrinone (Inocor) | 5-10 mcg/kg/min | 12 mcg/kg/min | 100 mg/100 mL NS | 1000 mcg/mL |
| dobutamine (Dobutrex) | 2.5-10 mcg/kg/min | 40 mcg/kg/min | 500 mg/250 mL D5W | 2000 mcg/mL |
| dopamine (Intropin) | 1-20 mcg/kg/min | <50 mcg/kg/min | 400 mg/250 mL D5W | 1600 mcg/mL |
| esmolol (Brevibloc) | 50-200 mcg/kg/min | 300 mcg/kg/min | 5 Gm/500 mL D5W | 10,000 mcg/mL |
| nitroprusside (Nipride) | 0.5-10 mcg/kg/min | 10 mcg/kg/min | 50 mg/250 mL D5W | 200 mcg/mL |

T J Designs • 1237 Laguna Lane • San Luis Obispo, CA 93405

### Pocket Guide C